MEDITATION FOR FAST LOSS WEIGHT

30 day challange to end emotional eating. Guided meditation to help you control hunger and release stress. Guided affirmation to achieve your weight goals forever

Dr. Nathan Stone

Copyright & Disclaimers

* **Author's note**: Please be aware that I am not certified health medical professional and I take no liability or responsibility for anything you decide to do because of the information in this book. This book is for meditation on how you can use meditation for weight loss. purpose exclusively. It is recommended that you talk to a health professional before making any significant changes to your diet or activity levels.

Table Of Content

INTRODUCTION TO MEDITATION FOR FAST LOSS WEIGHT

Reflection is a training that assists with interfacing the brain and body to accomplish a feeling of quiet. Individuals have been reflecting for a great many years as a profound practice. Today, numerous individuals use contemplation to lessen pressure and become increasingly mindful of their considerations.

There are numerous kinds of reflection. Some depend on the utilization of explicit expressions called mantras. Others center on breathing or keeping the brain right now.

These techniques can assist you with building up a superior comprehension of yourself, including how your brain and body functions.

This expanded mindfulness makes contemplation a valuable apparatus for better understanding your dietary patterns, which could bring about weight reduction. Peruse on to become familiar with the advantages of contemplation for weight reduction and how to begin.

What are the advantages of reflection for weight reduction?

Reflection won't cause you to get thinner medium-term. Be that as it may, with a little practice, it can conceivably effectsly affect your weight, yet in addition your idea designs.

Maintainable weight reduction

Contemplation is connected to an assortment of advantages. As far as weight reduction, care contemplation is by all accounts the most accommodating. A 2017 audit of existing examinations found that care contemplation was a compelling strategy for getting in shape and changing dietary patterns.

Care Contemplation Includes Giving Close Consideration To:

- where you are

- what you're doing

- how you're feeling right now

During care reflection, you'll recognize these viewpoints without judgment. Attempt to regard your activities and considerations as simply those — nothing else. Consider what you're feeling and doing, yet do whatever it takes not to order anything as being positive or negative. This gets simpler with normal practice.

Rehearsing care reflection can prompt long haul benefits, as well. Contrasted with different health food nuts, those rehearsing care are bound to keep the weight off, as per the 2017 audit.

Less blame and disgrace

Care reflection can be especially useful in controlling enthusiastic and stress-related eating. By getting progressively mindful of your considerations and feelings, you can perceive those occasions when you eat on the grounds that you're focused, as opposed to hungry.

It's likewise a decent apparatus to keep you from falling into the unsafe winding of disgrace and blame that a few people succumb to when attempting to change their dietary patterns. Care contemplation includes perceiving the truth about your sentiments and practices, without making a decision about you.

This urges you to excuse yourself for committing errors, for example, stress-eating a pack of potato chips. That pardoning can likewise keep you from catastrophizing, which is an extravagant term for what happens when you choose to arrange a pizza since you as of now "messed up" by eating a sack of chips.

How Might I Begin Contemplating For Weight Reduction?

Anybody with a psyche and body can rehearse contemplation. There's no requirement for any exceptional hardware or costly classes. For some, the hardest part is basically finding the time. Attempt to begin with something sensible, for example, 10 minutes per day or even every other day.

Ensure you approach a peaceful spot during these 10 minutes. In the event that you have kids, you might need to crush it in before they wake up or after they hit the hay to limit interruption. You can even have a go at doing it in the shower.

When you're in a tranquil spot, make yourself agreeable. You can sit or rests in any position that feels simple.

Start by concentrating on your breath, viewing your chest or stomach as it rises and falls. Feel the air as it moves all through your mouth or nose. Tune in to the sounds the air makes. Do this for a moment or two, until you begin to feel increasingly loose.

Next, With Your Eyes Open Or Shut, Follow These Means:

- Take a full breath in. Hold it for a few seconds.

- Gradually breathe out and rehash.

- Inhale normally.

Watch your breath as it enters your noses, raises your chest, or moves your gut, yet don't change it in any capacity.

Keep concentrating on your breath for 5 to 10 minutes.

You'll discover your brain meandering, which is totally typical. Simply recognize that your brain has meandered and return your consideration regarding your breath.

As you begin to wrap up, ponder how effectively your psyche meandered. At that point, recognize that it was so natural to take your consideration back to your breath.

Attempt to do this a larger number of days of the week than not. Remember that it probably won't feel extremely viable the initial barely any occasions you do it. Be that as it may, with customary practice, it'll get simpler and begin to feel progressively regular.

Where Would I Be Able To Discover Guided Contemplations?

In case you're interested about difficult different sorts of reflection or simply need some direction; you can discover an assortment of guided contemplations on the web. Remember that you don't really need to tail one that is intended for weight reduction.

While picking a guided contemplation on the web, attempt to avoid those promising medium-term results or offering trance.

Here's a guided care reflection from therapist Tara Brach, PhD, to kick you off.

You can likewise attempt these reflection applications. Different care procedures

Here are a couple of different tips to assist you with adopting a care based strategy to weight reduction:

Hinder your suppers. Concentrate on biting gradually and perceiving the flavor of each chomp.

Locate the opportune time to eat. Abstain from eating in a hurry or while performing multiple tasks.

Figure out how to perceive yearning and totality. In the event that you aren't ravenous, don't eat. In case you're full, don't continue onward. Attempt to tune in to what your body is letting you know.

Perceive how certain nourishments cause you to feel. Attempt to focus on how you feel in the wake of eating certain nourishments. Which ones cause you to feel tired? Which ones cause you to feel stimulated?

Excuse yourself. You believed that half quart of frozen yogurt would cause you to feel better, however it didn't. That is OK. Gain from it and proceed onward.

Settle on progressively attentive nourishment decisions. Invest more energy considering what you will eat before really eating.

Notice your longings. Longing for chocolate once more? Recognizing your desires can assist you with opposing them.

CHAPTER 1

WHAT IS MEDITATION WEIGHT LOSS

WEIGHT LOSS MEDICATION OR MEDITATION

Losing weight is a good thing. Some people try the diet, exercise, and medication for this purpose. Others will try yoga, meditation, and Chinese traditional methods to lose weight. In both ways, it is a good approach because we will get the same desired results.

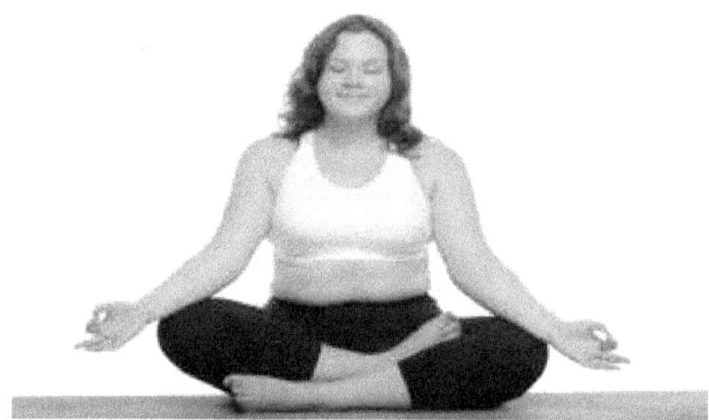

Is it possible to lose weight with meditation? Is it possible to lose weight with meditation? This article is not in favor of medications or meditation. I have watched people losing weight with yoga and meditation. Yoga helps you get in shape and it burns 2 to 3 calories per minute.

The best yoga exercise is "Ashtanga Vinyasa yoga" where there is never any separation between your breaths and movements. Every pose starts with inhales and ends on exhales. That is why yoga has good effects on n your metabolic rate. Yoga is also a good cardiovascular exercise.

Chinese traditional methods are also used to lose weight. Most people get good results with these methods and that is why Chinese tea, Chinese pills, and Chinese acupuncture are famous among people.

Meditation is not a method to lose weight but it is used to calm your mind and body. Meditation removes stress and it is a good way to release tension.

Medications are also successful for weight loss but there is a lot of discussion on this topic. It is always preferred to lose weight with diet and exercise. Medication cannot be a substitute for a healthy lifestyle. Healthy lifestyle guarantees long life and success. Meditation and yoga are indications of a good lifestyle.

Yoga or meditation can be used only if you are not overweight. If you are overweight, medications are necessary.

Medication Vs. Meditation

- You cannot use the medication without the consent of your doctor. Do not take risk of your life. Weight loss supplements, pills, and shakes are included in medications.

- Meditation can be done on your own. You can also use Chinese methods. Do not use acupuncture as a weight loss technique without medical supervision.

- Medications have some side effects while meditation has none.

- Medication makes you feel ill and sick. Yoga and meditation are indications of a good lifestyle.

- Chinese tea and other natural supplements improve your overall health while medicines are used for treatments of certain problems.

What Should Be Your Choice?

It depends on your health. If you are an overweight person, go with medication. If you are living a healthy life, do meditate for 15 minutes. It will make your life happy and peaceful.

How To Introduce Meditation In Your Life?

Most people do not have time to meditate. That is a problem. When we are living a healthy life, we do not pay attention to our fitness. Select a time and room where you will not be disturbed or interrupted. Go to your room and do meditation for 15 minutes. No more no less. Do not do it for more than 15 minutes for your 1st 10 days. I want you to stick with this plan. If you will spend more time in it you will not be able to find time for it.

Meditation and yoga are two different things. However, their purpose is single-minded devotion. These exercises develop focus, stability, and inner peace.

Easy Weight Loss For Women

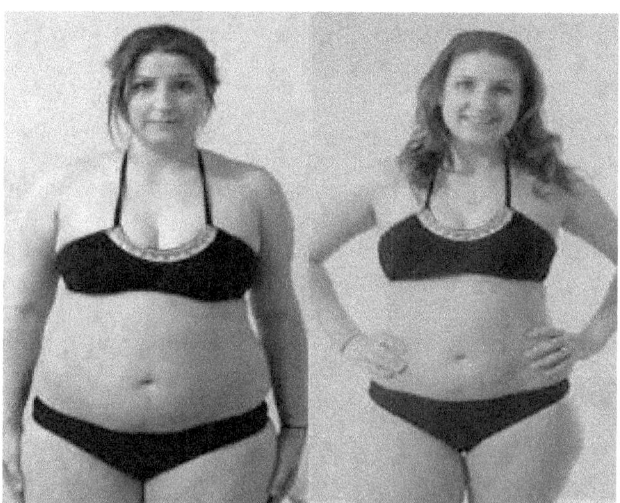

First things first ladies! Probably the first thing and greatest tip I have is to learn patience. Most of us do not even have the slightest idea of how much patience is required when it comes to dieting. Most of us fall into a program hoping all will go well if I follow this program slash diet for the next say week...

Well, this is exactly why I am putting this list of tips together for you to see what exactly is required when starting a new weight loss program.

❖   **MEDITATION**

Start with learning to meditate. In meditation, there is an absolute essence of patience and this will also learn you to be comfortable with your body. It will also decrease those stress levels that have been proven to help you peel on the Pounds. Meditation will teach you durability and the needed endurance to complete the weight loss program and not stop when you have reached a certain stage.

❖   **LIFT HEAVY WEIGHTS**

Now you might feel that you don't want to lift heavy weights because you do not want to build muscle. The truth of the matter is that when we lift heavy weights, our diet mainly regulates if we will build bulky muscles or tone our flabby bits. So please understand this correctly, lift heavy weights only if you are following a strict eating plan. Remember to do the workout in such a way that you get a proper cardio-effect from the weight training as well.

A proper heavyweight training exercise would be one where you do a proper circuit and move quickly between exercises so you don't have any extended periods of rest.

This will increase cardio-effect and minimize bulk.

So what are we talking about here? Basically circuit weight training with big body movements. This will include exercises such as squats, lunges, chest presses, pull-ups, shoulder presses and other affiliated exercises that will get a large number of muscles active and really ramp up your metabolism. This will ensure fat loss without bulking.

What makes this Weight Loss For Women tip so attractive, is that if you are not yet comfortable with your body, as most women that feel overweight are, you might feel to do these exercises in the comfort of your own home.

❖   **RECHECK YOUR DIET**

A healthy diet is not the same as a fat loss diet. You might be eating healthy foods such as grains, nuts, etc. Although they are high in fiber and packed with vitamins they also have high sugar content. A better alternative would be to replace the grain in your diet with fruits and veg. Try to steer clear of high GI fruits such as Watermelon, Pineapple, and Banana to name a few.

CHAPTER 2

WHAT IS EMOTIONAL EATING

We don't generally eat just to fulfill physical appetite. A considerable lot of us additionally go to nourishment for comfort, stress help, or to compensate ourselves. What's more, when we do, we will in general reach for lousy nourishment, desserts, and other consoling however undesirable nourishments.

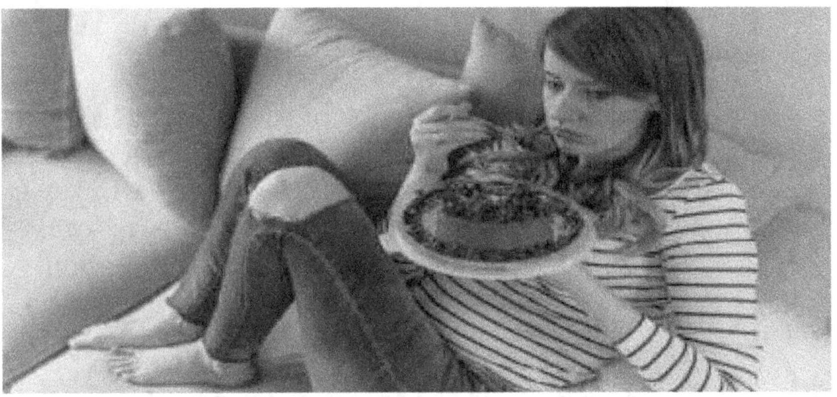

You may go after a 16 ounces of frozen yogurt when you're feeling down, request a pizza in case you're exhausted or desolate, or swing by the drive-through following a distressing day busy working. Enthusiastic eating is utilizing nourishment to cause yourself to feel better—to fill passionate requirements, as opposed to your stomach. Sadly, enthusiastic eating doesn't fix passionate issues. Truth be told, it for the most part aggravates you feel. A while later, not exclusively does the first intense subject matter remain, yet you likewise feel regretful for gorging.

- It is safe to say that you are an enthusiastic eater?

- Do you eat more when you're feeling focused?

- Do you eat when you're not eager or when you're full?

- Improve (to quiet and calm yourself when you're dismal, frantic, exhausted, on edge, and so forth.)?

- Do you reward yourself with nourishment?

- Do you consistently eat until you've stuffed yourself?

- Does nourishment cause you to feel safe? Do you feel like nourishment is a companion?

- Do you feel feeble or crazy around nourishment?

The enthusiastic eating cycle

Periodically utilizing nourishment as a jolt of energy, a prize, or to celebrate isn't really an awful thing. Be that as it may, when eating is your essential passionate method for dealing with stress—when your first motivation is to open the fridge at whatever point you're focused on, agitated, irate, forlorn, depleted, or exhausted—you stall out in an unfortunate cycle where the genuine inclination or issue is rarely tended to.

Passionate appetite can't be loaded up with nourishment. Eating may feel great at the time, yet the emotions that set off the eating are still there. Also, you frequently feel more terrible than you did before in view of the superfluous calories you've quite recently devoured. You beat yourself for failing and not having more resolution.

Intensifying the issue, you quit learning more advantageous approaches to manage your feelings, you have an increasingly hard time controlling your weight, and you feel progressively weak over both nourishment and your sentiments. However, regardless of how frail you feel over nourishment and your sentiments, it is conceivable to roll out a positive improvement. You can learn more advantageous approaches to manage your feelings, dodge triggers, overcome longings, lastly shut down enthusiastic eating.

The Distinction Between Passionate Yearning And Physical Appetite

Before you can break liberated from the pattern of enthusiastic eating, you first need to figure out how to recognize passionate and physical yearning. This can be trickier than it sounds, particularly on the off chance that you routinely use nourishment to manage your emotions.

Passionate craving can be amazing, so it's anything but difficult to confuse it with physical yearning. In any case, there are signs you can search for to assist you with differentiating physical and passionate appetite.

Enthusiastic craving goes ahead out of nowhere. It hits you in a moment and feels overpowering and earnest. Physical appetite, then again, goes ahead more bit by bit. The desire to eat doesn't feel as critical or request moment fulfillment (except if you haven't eaten for an exceptionally prolonged stretch of time).

Passionate yearning desires explicit solace nourishments. At the point when you're genuinely eager, nearly anything sounds great—including solid stuff like vegetables. In any case, passionate appetite longs for shoddy nourishment or sugary tidbits that give a moment surge. You sense that you need cheesecake or pizza, and everything else should be ignored.

Passionate craving regularly prompts careless eating. Before you know it, you've eaten an entire sack of chips or a whole 16 ounces of dessert without truly focusing or completely getting a charge out of it. At the point when you're eating in light of physical yearning, you're ordinarily increasingly mindful of what you're doing.

Passionate craving isn't fulfilled once you're full. You continue needing to an ever increasing extent, regularly eating until you're awkwardly stuffed. Physical appetite, then again, shouldn't be full.

You feel fulfilled when your stomach is full.

Passionate craving isn't situated in the stomach. As opposed to a snarling tummy or an ache in your stomach, you feel your appetite as a hankering you can't escape your head. You're centered on explicit surfaces, tastes, and scents.

Enthusiastic yearning frequently prompts lament, blame, or disgrace. At the point when you eat to fulfill physical yearning, you're probably not going to feel regretful or embarrassed in light of the fact that you're just giving your body what it needs. On the off chance that you feel remorseful after you eat, it's presumable on the grounds that you realize where it counts that you're not eating for wholesome reasons.

- **Enthusiastic appetite versus Physical appetite**

Enthusiastic appetite goes ahead suddenly   Physical hunger goes ahead bit by bit

Enthusiastic appetite feels like it should be fulfilled instantly   Physical yearning can pause

Enthusiastic appetite longs for explicit solace foods Physical hunger is available to alternatives—bunches of things sound great

Enthusiastic appetite isn't happy with a full stomach.   Physical hunger stops when you're full

Enthusiastic eating triggers sentiments of blame, feebleness, and shame Eating to fulfill physical appetite doesn't cause you to feel awful about yourself

- **Distinguish Your Passionate Eating Triggers**

The initial phase in ending passionate eating is distinguishing your own triggers. What circumstances, spots, or emotions make you go after the solace of nourishment? Most enthusiastic eating is connected to upsetting sentiments, yet it can likewise be activated by positive feelings, for example, remunerating you for accomplishing an objective or praising an occasion or upbeat occasion.

- **Basic Reasons For Enthusiastic Eating**

Stress – Ever notice how pressure makes you hungry? It's not simply in your brain. At the point when stress is ceaseless, as it so frequently is in our confused, quick paced world, your body delivers significant levels of the pressure hormone, cortisol. Cortisol triggers desires for salty, sweet, and singed nourishments—nourishments that give you an eruption of vitality and joy. The more uncontrolled worry in your life, the more probable you are to go to nourishment for enthusiastic help.

Stuffing feelings – Eating can be an approach to incidentally quietness or "stuff down" awkward feelings, including outrage, dread, misery, nervousness, forlornness, disdain, and disgrace. While you're desensitizing yourself with nourishment, you can maintain a strategic distance from the troublesome feelings you'd preferably not feel.

Weariness or sentiments of vacancy – Do you ever eat basically to give yourself something to do, to diminish fatigue, or as an approach to fill a void in your life? You feel unfulfilled and void, and nourishment is an approach to possess your mouth and your time. At the time, it tops you off and diverts you from basic sentiments of purposelessness and disappointment with your life.

Youth propensities – Think back to your beloved recollections of nourishment. Did your folks reward great conduct with frozen yogurt, take you out for pizza when you got a decent report card, or serve you desserts when you were feeling pitiful? These propensities can frequently extend into adulthood. Or then again your eating might be driven by sentimentality—for appreciated recollections of barbecuing burgers in the lawn with your father or preparing and eating treats with your mother.

Social impacts – Getting together with others for a supper is an incredible method to ease pressure, however it can likewise prompt indulging. It's anything but difficult to enjoy basically in light of the fact that the nourishment is there or on the grounds that every other person is eating. You may likewise indulge in social circumstances out of anxiety. Or on the other hand maybe your family or friend network urges you to gorge, and it's simpler to oblige the gathering.

- **Keep An Enthusiastic Eating Journal**

You most likely perceived yourself in at any rate a couple of the past portrayals. Be that as it may, all things considered, you'll need to get considerably progressively explicit. Perhaps the most ideal approaches to recognize the examples behind your enthusiastic eating is to keep track with a nourishment and temperament journal.

Each time you indulge or feel constrained to go after your rendition of solace nourishment Kryptonite, pause for a minute to make sense of what set off the inclination. On the off chance that you backtrack, you'll ordinarily locate an upsetting occasion that kicked of the passionate eating cycle. Record it all in your nourishment and state of mind journal: what you ate (or needed to eat), what happened to agitate you, how you felt before you ate, what you felt as you were eating, and how you felt a short time later.

After some time, you'll see an example develop. Perhaps you generally wind up pigging out yourself in the wake of investing energy with a basic companion. Or on the other hand maybe you stress eat at whatever point you're on a cutoff time or when you go to family works. When you recognize your passionate eating triggers, the subsequent stage is distinguishing more beneficial approaches to take care of your emotions.

Find Different Approaches To Take Care Of Your Sentiments

In the event that you don't have a clue how to deal with your feelings in a manner that doesn't include nourishment, you won't have the option to control your dietary patterns for long. Diets so frequently come up short since they offer intelligent wholesome exhortation which possibly works on the off chance that you have cognizant power over your dietary patterns. It doesn't work when feelings commandeer the procedure, requesting a prompt result with nourishment.

So as to stop passionate eating, you need to discover different approaches to satisfy yourself inwardly. It's insufficient to comprehend the pattern of passionate eating or even to comprehend your triggers, in spite of the fact that that is an enormous initial step. You need options in contrast to nourishment that you can go to for passionate satisfaction.

- **Options In Contrast To Passionate Eating**

In case you're discouraged or forlorn, call somebody who consistently causes you to feel better, play with your canine or feline, or take a gander at a most loved photograph or treasured keepsake.

In case you're restless, exhaust your anxious vitality by moving to your main tune, crushing a pressure ball, or going for a lively stroll.

In case you're depleted, treat yourself with a hot cup of tea, clean up, light some scented candles, or enclose yourself by a warm cover.

In case you're exhausted, perused a decent book, watch a parody appear, investigate the outside, or go to a movement you appreciate (carpentry, playing the guitar, shoot.

Benefit Of Meditation Weight Loss

Your endeavors around practicing and eating admirably are helping your circulatory strain and your weight. Something different may likewise support: contemplation.

Reflection - the act of concentrating so as to discover quiet and lucidity - can bring down hypertension. It can likewise assist you with overseeing pressure, which drives a few people to eat.

"Individuals regularly put on weight from attempting to comfort themselves with nourishment," says Adam Perlman, MD, official chief of Duke Integrative Medicine.

Despite the fact that there's not a ton of research demonstrating that contemplation legitimately causes you get in shape, reflection helps you become progressively mindful of your musings and activities, including those that identify with nourishment.

For instance, an exploration audit indicated that contemplation can help with both gorging and enthusiastic eating.

Step By Step Instructions To Quiet Your Mind

Do you think that its difficult to close down the gab, clear your head, or discover a feeling of quiet? These methods could help. What's more, they may have different advantages, as well.

"Any approach to turn out to be progressively careful will control that procedure," Perlman says.

Step By Step Instructions To Meditate

There are numerous approaches to reflect. The CDC says that most kinds of contemplation share these four things for all intents and purpose:

A calm area. You can pick where to ruminate - your preferred seat? On a walk? It's up to you.

A particular agreeable stance, for example, sitting, resting, standing, or strolling.

A focal point of consideration. You can concentrate on a word or expression, your breath, or something different.

An open disposition. It's not unexpected to have different considerations while you ruminate. Make an effort not to get excessively keen on those contemplations. Hold taking your consideration back to your breath, expression, or whatever else it is you're concentrating on.

Pick the spot, time, and strategy that you need to attempt. You can likewise take a class to get familiar with the nuts and bolts.

Turning into a 'Witness,' Not a Judge

Contemplating requires a pledge to stop and search inside and around you, regardless of whether you have just a couple of seconds, says Geneen Roth, creator of the New York Times success Women Food and God.

"The manner in which I show reflection and incorporate it for myself is to concentrate on being an observer to your considerations and less to what extent you have to rehearse," Roth says. "You need to figure out how to calm your mind and some of the time stay away from the accounts you let yourself know, similar to you have to go eat treats or that sack of chips."

Advantages Of Meditation Weight Loss

At this point, you've presumably taken a stab at everything to shed off those bothersome pounds, from limiting your calories to strengthening your exercise schedule. While these endeavors may be helping you shed a pound or two at regular intervals, there's something that can give you that additional lift: contemplation.

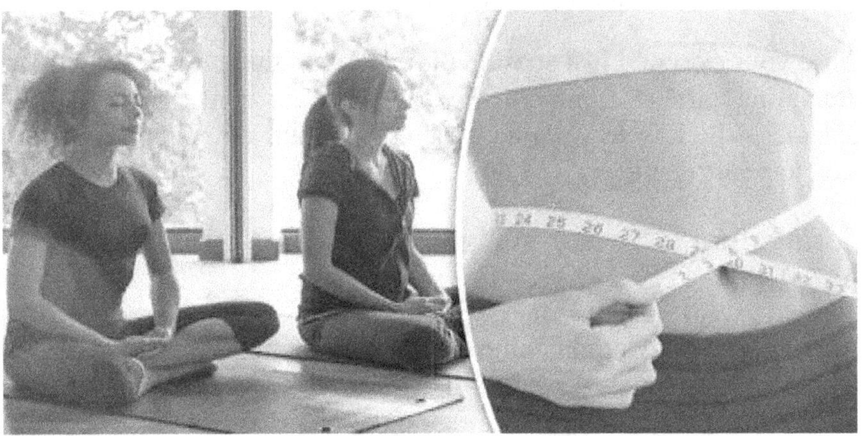

This sans cost, characteristic, basic system can be extremely successful in helping you thin down, while likewise lightening pressure and nervousness. The examination encompassing careful reflection rehearses proposes that contemplation is firmly connected to weight reduction.

The ideas of care and contemplation cannot just lower your feelings of anxiety and lift mindfulness. Having a mindful psyche can keep you from voraciously consuming food and passionate eating. Along these lines, contemplation for weight reduction can be a normally sound and viable approach to get thinner and eat better.

Basically, contemplation is the demonstration of concentrating on getting increasingly careful. As indicated by the American Meditation Society, during contemplation, an individual's consideration basically streams inwards as opposed to taking part in the external universe of movement. The training includes freeing the psyche with the point from coming back to a condition of quiet feelings and clear reasoning.

A few people practice reflection for just five minutes per day, however specialists recommending attempting to stir that up to around 20 minutes per day. For those who're simply beginning, consider taking five minutes soon after you wake up to clear your psyche before continuing ahead with your day.

Close your eyes and just spotlight on your breathing example without attempting to transform it. On the off chance that your psyche meander, which is very regular when beginning, simply controls it back to your relaxing.

Connection Between Weight Loss And Meditation Lose Weight

The primary motivation behind why contemplation can be so viable in helping individuals get more fit is that it adjusts the cognizant and the oblivious brain into concurring on the progressions that you need to apply to your practices. These progressions incorporate directing longings for unfortunate nourishments, changing dietary patterns, and finding the inspiration to work out.

Editorial manager's Picks

- Is Breathing Essential Oils from Portable Diffusers Safer Than Vamping?

- Is Breathing Essential Oils from Portable Diffusers Safer Than Vamping?

- To an ever increasing extent, individuals are choosing for utilize basic oil diffusers as an option in contrast to vamping. Basic oils are more beneficial

Sinusitis: Top 8 Essential Oils for Relief

Sinusitis—a contamination or aggravation of the sinuses—is an unfathomably regular affliction.1 Often brought about by sensitivities or sickness, sinus irritation results […]

Top 20 Essential Oils For Relieving Pain And Inflammation

It is safe to say that you are in torment? Everybody encounters a throbbing painfulness sporadically. Some uneasiness is mellow and bearable. Did you realize that […]

It's consequently imperative to have the brain associated with your weight reduction venture since it's the place the hurtful, weight-picking up propensities including passionate eating are settled in. Contemplation in a perfect world encourages you become progressively mindful of these propensities and musings, conquer them with time, and even supplant them with positive, sound propensities.

Building up a contemplation routine will likewise assist you with keeping weight reduction alive. It basically carries the item to the front line of your psyche and your day. Along these lines, it's a lot harder to overlook, which it will persuade you to continue onward.

Reflection makes a more elevated level of fixation and spotlights on your weight reduction objectives. Since it's so natural to get diverted, removing some time from your bustling day to reflect will harbor that inspiration.

Mental Well-Being

Reflection and care have likewise been appeared to improve mental wellbeing. Care has been appeared to bring down passionate eating, voraciously consuming food, and for the most part improve the weight reduction process.

Stress help is perhaps the quickest advantage of contemplation. It basically removes you from the battle or-flight mode by bringing down the degrees of stress hormones in your body. Stress hormones, for example, cortisol normally signal the body to store more calories as fat. Along these lines, high cortisol levels are going to make it much hard for you to shed additional weight, regardless of whether you're reliably settling on sound decisions.

As indicated by an examination directed via Carnegie Mellon University, everything necessary is around 25 minutes of reflection three days straight to lessen pressure significantly.1 In another 2016 investigation, members demonstrated expanded unwinding, consideration, mind-body mindfulness, smoothness, and even cerebrum movement subsequent to finishing a couple of short contemplation sessions.2 The examination additionally expressed that degrees of restraint could increment with day by day contemplation practice.

At last, in an ongoing examination audit, analysts assessed that the job of contemplation on weight reduction, alongside the practices that are frequently connected with poor eating.3 They presumed that careful reflection could be useful in diminishing the recurrence of voraciously consuming food and passionate eating.

Care

Despite the fact that care is very not the same as contemplation, the two ideas go connected at the hip. Reflection causes you let go of things to come and past. Maybe you have had various bombed endeavors at weight reduction previously or you're encountering a few nerves about the future, for example, disposing of poor propensities. Care while thinking lets you appreciate the present without focusing a lot on these stressors.

The Most Effective Method To Ensure That Meditation For Weight Loss Works For You Pick The Right Practice

There are various distinctive contemplation styles that you can go with, however they all follow a comparative essential method of quieting the brain and setting aside some effort to inhale and getting mindful of the current minute. It's savvy to attempt various strategies that sound fascinating to you to discover which ones work best.

Think About Aromatherapy

Fragrance based treatment has additionally been demonstrated viable in quieting the body, which is useful when meditating.4 you can for the most part use fragrance based treatment for contemplation in two distinct manners. The first is diffusing the oil into the air.

This can be useful in advancing unwinding, invigorating the faculties, and making an encompassing space where you can truly center. On the other hand, take a stab at utilizing basic oils in an individual fragrance based treatment diffuser like Zen, Vibrant, Active, or Healthy MONQ. Tenderly inhale MONQ into your mouth and afterward out through your nose. MONQ ought not to be breathed in into the lungs.

Also, basic oils can be applied topically to the skin after weakening with transporter oil.

CHAPTER 3

GUIDED MEDITATION VS UNGUIDED MEDITATION

As the prominence of reflection develops, more individuals are posing the inquiry should I learn guided or unguided contemplation.

I needed to compose this article to give you a diagram of the advantages, contrasts and weaknesses of both of these contemplation styles.

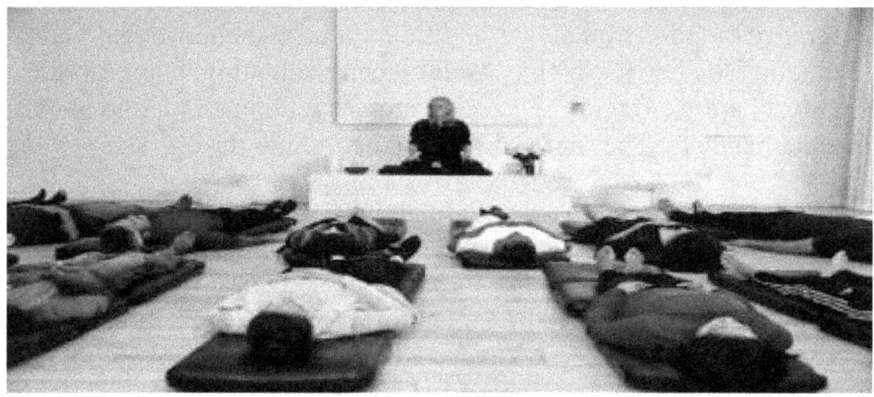

Guided reflection is driven by an educator, who guides you bit by bit through your contemplation classes or by means of online sound. Unguided contemplation is polished without outer guidelines. Rather, you lead yourself through your own contemplations. For the most part guided reflection is utilized to support tenderfoots and unguided contemplation is a venturing stone for further developed mediators.

Guided Meditation Or Unguided Meditation

Guided Meditation is an extraordinary beginning stage for novices who want to contemplate just because.

In Guided reflection your instructor will lead you through the contemplation practice from beginning to end. The educator will guide you where to take your consideration. At the point when your brain meanders the instructor will urge you to pull together however your contemplation ventures?

"I'm a significant psychotic scholar, truly an adrenalized individual. In any case, after contemplation, I felt this delightful peacefulness and benevolent association."

Guided contemplation is the ideal method to get into a daily practice and propensity. This is essential in the event that you need to develop consistency and begin to see the advantages of contemplation in your life.

Many guided reflections will include a bit by bit method for learning and rehearsing contemplation, with the goal that you can gradually manufacture your certainty.

Guided reflections can be led week by week at neighborhood contemplation focus or day by day by means of application sound CD or on the web.

Some first-time meditators discover the help of a neighborhood class helps enormously with their reflection practice. During the classes amateurs can pose inquiries from the educator and furthermore hear different disappointments that individual mediators are having in their every day practice.

❖   **DISAPPOINTMENT**

Apprentices regularly find pondering baffling on the off chance that they're attempting to go only it at home. Guided contemplation is the most ideal approach to keep your reflection on target and moving the correct way.

The issue with contemplating alone is you can wind up going here and there aimlessly, and not know whether you're doing any acceptable whatsoever or burning through your time. Having an expert teacher can assist with guaranteeing that you don't feel like your endeavors are silly.

❖ **BIT BY BIT**

It's unbelievably essential to have a bit by bit plan when you first beginning contemplating. As this can reduce any diverting, and letting your contemplation head ruinous way.

A decent guided contemplation plan won't toss you in the profound end without a lifejacket. It will let you squirm your toes in the water first. At that point gradually move you into the shallows until you feel progressively sure.

Attempt This Short 5 Minute Guided Meditation

❖ **LENGTH**

An expert teacher will begin by acquainting learners with short meetings. These can be as little as 30 second as long as 10 minutes.

This little length of reflection can assist you with building little additions of focus.

Proficient mediators can ponder as long as 10 hours in addition to every day.

At the point when you are simply starting a brief reflection can feel like an unending length of time. The mystery is consistency and the more you practice each day, the more you'll have the option to ruminate.

❖ **REFLECTION FLOW**

Guided Meditation permits you to adhere to the directions of your instructor without losing your reflection stream.

As amateurs you have to put all your consideration on watching and remaining present in your reflection.

In case you're attempting unguided contemplation you may discover your consideration is part between attempting to center and endeavoring to direct yourself. Numerous individuals lean toward guided reflection, so they can concentrate on what's significant. This permits them to quit agonizing over whether they're hitting the nail on the head, to what extent they ought to reflect or where they ought to center.

"It feels better. Kinda like when you need to close your PC down, just now and then when it goes insane, you simply shut it down and when you turn it on, it's alright once more. That is the thing that reflection is to me." One of the rewards about guided reflection is there is an assortment of nearby instructors and online trainings.

As reflection turns out to be progressively well known, there are an ever increasing number of instructors surfacing everywhere throughout the Internet. This implies you have a buffet of instructors that you can interface with and gain from.

There are additionally various phenomenal reflection applications for advanced cells. This is an incredible method for figuring out how to think at home and getting support from their bit by bit programs.

Numerous tenderfoots despite everything love going to contemplation classes at their nearby studios. Contemplating with others can expand the force of your reflection and can rouse you to proceed with when you want to surrender.

❖   **PICKING UP CONFIDENCE**

The most significant thing about contemplation is that you keep your training predictable, one to 2 times each day. Along these lines you are picking up certainty and developing in your capacity to reflect.

As novices isn't shrewd to begin unguided contemplation all alone, as this can prompt overpowering dissatisfaction. The more disappointed you get with an unstructured reflection plan, the simpler it is to simply say you'll do it tomorrow.

In the issue with doing it tomorrow, is that can transform into one week from now, one month from now or one year from now.

The explanation guided contemplation work so well, is it gives you an educator to gain from, set term and an organized bit by bit plan.

❖   **GOING SOLO**

The intensity of unguided contemplation is that you can take advantage of your inward intensity of quietness and stillness.

The priests, who ponder more than 10 hours in addition to every day, utilize unguided contemplation to rest their psyche, recuperate their bodies and discover illumination.

❖   **THE TIGHTROPE**

Unguided contemplation can resemble navigating a precarious situation. On the off chance that you don't have the foggiest idea how to adjust, you may fall into the reasoning that reflection is simply to hard. The perils of rehearsing unguided contemplation to ahead of schedule, is it can lead you to overpower, dissatisfaction and disillusionment.

Numerous apprentices, who attempt unguided contemplation, are not sufficiently able to hold they center object and constantly become involved with the surge of approaching musings.

You have a huge number of musings daily. Your considerations can resemble the hare gap in Alice in Wonderland. One idea can prompt another, to another, until out of nowhere you are miles from the absolute previously thought. In unguided reflection you are your own contemplation manage. This implies you have to pick your center article and during the contemplation if your psyche begins to meander, you are liable for taking your brain back to center.

It's significant you develop some fundamental establishment in center and focus before you attempt unguided contemplation. The general purpose to utilizing guided reflection practice first, is to locate a reliable stream every day.

Since the advantages from reflection originate from consistency!

Moving from guided reflections to unguided contemplation is a characteristic stream and it's the most ideal path for new novices.

Guided reflection gives you a strong establishment for your contemplation practice. Unguided contemplation is utilized to amplify and develop your reflection venture. Quiet reflection is like an unguided contemplation. This style of reflection you utilize a center item like your breath, an envision object or a quiet mantra.

Quiet reflection is an amazing method to connect with your inward stillness.

At the point when you practice quiet reflection you open an inner space, where you can discover revival, harmony and edification.

Why Meditation Is Good Than Others Weight Loss

With regards to eating and dealing with our weight and our wellbeing, it is imperative to recognize the significance of the psyche body association. Our chaotic, jam-stuffed lives may truly be overloading us. In an ongoing survey, 38% of grown-ups announced eating or indulging in the previous month as a way to manage or maintain a strategic distance from pressure, and about half of these grown-ups detailed these practices in the previous week.

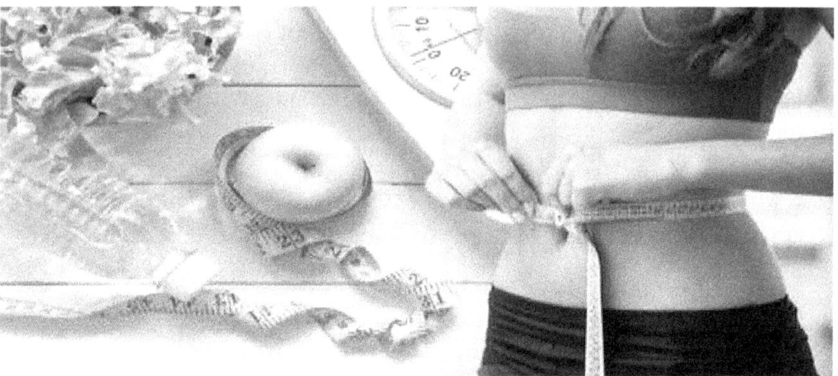

On the off chance that this is an inclination or conduct you can identify with, you're not the only one. The uplifting news is: There are steps you can take that might have the option to assist you with managing or get more fit, and contemplation for weight reduction is one of them.

Explicit practices and procedures — reflection, careful eating, and instinctive eating — can assist us with learning or relearn how to have a solid relationship with nourishment and how to evacuate any dangerous sentiments we may have encompassing eating. Weight reduction might be a symptom of developing this restored relationship, yet it's significant not to build up getting in shape as the essential objective. Doing so may compel us with the goal that we can't genuinely eat naturally or in a careful manner.

Rather, center around getting a charge out of nourishments — eating since you're ravenous, not on the grounds that you're worried about work or family issues and feeling overpowered. You will learn through these practices how to acknowledge and cherish your body for everything it can accomplish for you.

With regards to discussing reflection for weight reduction or contemplation for eating and progressing in the direction of building up a sound connection with nourishment, it can assist with understanding what the wording implies.

Stress or passionate eating happens when individuals will in general eat and indulge as a result of compelling feelings or sentiments, as opposed to reacting to their own inward prompts of yearning. Here and there when we experience compelling feelings, these feelings can exceed our physical sentiments of completion and satiation, and this can bring about us gorging. In these cases, nourishment is utilized as a way of dealing with stress, dulling forceful feelings immediately. In any case, it's fundamental to recognize that this experience contributes toward sustaining a cycle. Feeling distressing feelings can prompt indulging, which prompts blame or disgrace, hovering back to feeling — and not having the option to process or handle — negative feelings or stress.

Careful eating is a procedure or system you can use to help fix your relationship with nourishment and eating encounters. It calls us to be available and to draw in our faculties — how the nourishment tastes, smells, and in particular, how it causes our bodies to feel. Careful eating joins natural eating, to assist us with easing back down and tune in to our inner prompts of genuine appetite versus signals of satiation, and in that capacity, it can assist us with lessening or even completely stop our passionate or voraciously consuming food.

While careful eating can prompt weight reduction, shedding pounds ought not to be the objective result or inspiration. In the event that our nourishment decisions are made dependent on a specific physical result we are wanting, it demonstrates that we have just quit eating carefully. The Headspace application incorporates a 30-meeting preparing pack as a total program to show careful eating.

Natural eating is a brain body, non-diet way to deal with wellbeing and health. It dismisses the idea of consuming fewer calories and instructs us to confide in our bodies and tune in to our inward physical signals, with the objective of mending our relationship with nourishment. Natural eating incorporates standards of careful eating; anyway it includes a more extensive extended way of thinking that ranges over, moving your body since it feels great to move, and utilizing nourishment data without predisposition.

How Reflection May Assist Us With Dealing With Our Weight

Similarly as reflection can assist us with stress, resting, center, and substantially more, it can likewise affect our relationship with eating and dealing with our weight.

With regards to getting thinner, we regularly consider taking a turn class or deciding on the serving of mixed greens rather than a burger for lunch. Thusly, it might appear to be illogical to think about sitting in one spot and centering your contemplations, and doing a reflection for weight reduction. These sorts of observations are just review some portion of the image. Remember that weight reduction isn't just physical, and it's not just highly contrasting. As people we're passionate creatures, and recognizing that reality is useful in building up a solid relationship with nourishment, and conceivably losing muscle versus fat or keeping up whatever weight is most advantageous for our bodies.

Consider a 2017 meta-examination of 19 unique investigations that found that run of the mill weight reduction techniques (diet and exercise) work temporarily, however in the long run the examination members' weight was recovered after the projects finished. Then again, weight reduction conventions that included care intercessions, for example, reflection (notwithstanding eating admirably and working out), apparently were increasingly viable in lessening weight and keeping it off among study members.

All in all, for what reason is it conceivable that reflection causes with regards to weight reduction, precisely? There are physical and mental variables influencing everything. Another 2017 meta-investigation found that summed up reflection diminished cortisol and C-responsive protein levels. In the event that our cortisol levels are reliably high, this is associated with the perseverance of corpulence after some time, as indicated by a recent report.

Mentally, explore shows that contemplation may help squash gorging. A 2014 survey analyzed 14 unique examinations and found that utilizing careful contemplation as the #1 intercession diminished voraciously consuming food and enthusiastic eating. Reflection has been appeared to bring down our feelings of anxiety. Indeed, Headspace lessens worry in 10 days. This is significant on the grounds that pressure is a contributing element, making a large number of us indulge. Reflection instructs us to sit with and watch our feelings without condemning, rather than depending on our go-to ways of dealing with stress like overindulging on nourishment.

5 Different Ways Contemplation Can Help Advance A Sound Connection With Eating

Reflection can assist us with turning out to be increasingly careful eaters and even location any passionate eating issues that may persevere.

1. Expel the disgrace and blame. For the individuals who battle with passionate eating, feeling focused can prompt indulging to mitigate or maintain a strategic distance from these sentiments. This can prompt blame or disgrace. Break the cycle. Contemplation not just decreases pressure, which evacuates the trigger in any case, yet it additionally causes you become increasingly mindful of your feelings and sentiments, so you can perceive those occasions when you're eating when focused on versus when you're really ravenous. Contemplation has additionally been appeared to build our sympathy, which may make us become all the more tolerating of others who may have distinctive body types from our own.

2. Keep up weight reduction and a sound load for the long stretch. Contemplation can help your weight reduction endeavors stick. While diet and exercise may assist you with arriving at your weight reduction objectives, reflection close by smart dieting and exercise puts forth weight reduction attempts manageable.

3. Lower pressure and aggravation levels. Reflection decreases cortisol and C-responsive protein levels, which is gainful to our general wellbeing and may assist us with accomplishing weight reduction and keep up a sound weight. Cortisol is related with putting away fat in our mid-region zone (gut fat), and raised C-receptive protein levels can be an indication of aggravation, which is at the foundation of numerous infections including heftiness.

4. Better control of yearnings. On the off chance that you battle with passionate or voraciously consuming food, it tends to be difficult to battle those extreme nourishment yearnings. Research shows that care contemplation can assist us with controlling passionate and voraciously consuming food.

5. Abatement our pressure and nervousness. Getting more fit requires a great deal of exertion, and keeping the weight off can be unpleasant, in any event, prompting sentiments of nervousness. Thirty days of utilizing the Headspace application for day by day contemplation lessens worry by a third, so it is a demonstrated apparatus.

CHAPTER 4

BEGINNERS GUIDE TO MEDITATION

Reflection has helped me to shape all my different propensities; it's helped me to turn out to be increasingly tranquil, progressively centered, less stressed over inconvenience, increasingly grateful and mindful to everything in my life. I'm a long way from great; however it has helped me made some amazing progress.

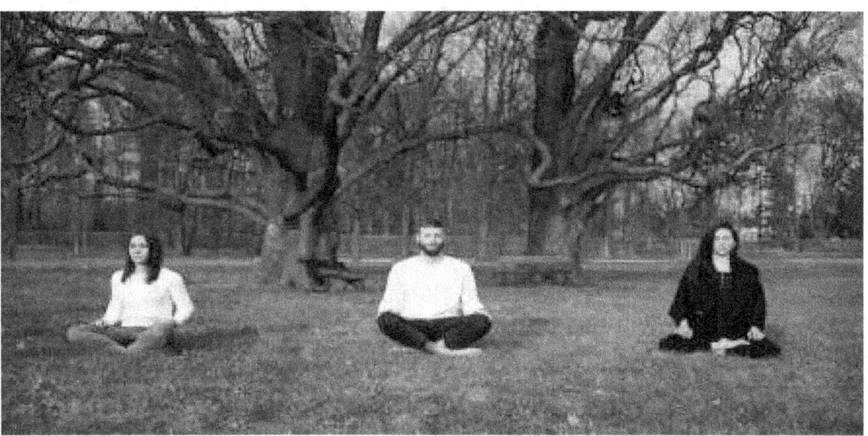

Presumably in particular, it has helped me comprehend my own psyche. Before I began contemplating, I never considered what was happening inside my head — it would simply occur, and I would follow its orders like a robot. Nowadays, the entirety of that despite everything occurs, except to an ever increasing extent, I am mindful of what's happening. I can settle on a decision about whether to follow the orders. I comprehend myself better (not totally, yet better), and that has given me expanded adaptability and opportunity.

So … I enthusiastically prescribe this propensity. And keeping in mind that I'm not saying it's simple, you can begin little and show signs of improvement and better as you practice. Try not to hope to be acceptable from the start — that is the reason it's designated "practice"!

These tips aren't planned for helping you to turn into a specialist …
they should assist you with beginning and continue onward. You
don't need to actualize them at the same time — attempt a couple,
return to this article, attempt a couple of something else.

Sit for only two minutes. This will appear to be absurdly simple, to
simply ruminate for two minutes. That is great. Start with only two
minutes per day for seven days. On the off chance that that works out
in a good way, increment by an additional two minutes and do that
for seven days. In the event that all works out in a good way, by
expanding only a little at once, you'll be ruminating for 10 minutes
every day in the second month, which is astounding! Yet, start little
first.

Do it first thing every morning. It's anything but difficult to state, "I'll
think each day," however then neglect to do it. Rather, set an update
for each morning when you get up, and put a note that says "think"
some place where you'll see it.

Try not to become involved with the how — simply do. A great
many people stress over where to sit, how to sit, what pad to utilize
… this is all pleasant, yet it isn't so critical to begin. Start just by
sitting on a seat, or on your lounge chair. Or then again on your bed.
In case you're agreeable on the ground, sit with folded legs. It's only
for two minutes from the outset at any rate, so simply sit. Later you
can stress over upgrading it so you'll be agreeable for more, yet
before all else it doesn't make a difference much, simply sit some
place peaceful and agreeable.

Check in with how you're feeling. As you first subside into your
reflection meeting, just verify how you're feeling. How does your
body feel? What is the nature of your psyche? Occupied? Tired?
Restless? See whatever you're bringing to this reflection meeting as
totally OK.

Tally your breaths. Since you're settled in, direct your concentration
toward your breath. Simply place the consideration on your breath as

it comes in, and finish it your nose right down to your lungs. Take a stab at tallying "one" as you take in the main breath, at that point "two" as you inhale out. Rehash this to the check of 10, at that point start again at one.

Return when you meander. Your brain will meander. This is a practically outright conviction. There's no issue with that. At the point when you notice your psyche meandering, grin, and just delicately come back to your breath. Check "one" once more, and begin once again. You may feel a little dissatisfaction, yet it's consummately OK to not remain centered, we as a whole do it. This is the training, and you won't be acceptable at it for a brief period.

Build up a caring disposition. At the point when you notice musings and emotions emerging during reflection, as they will, takes a gander at them with a cordial demeanor. Consider them to be companions, not interlopers or foes. They are a piece of you, however not every one of you. Be amicable and not cruel.

Try not to stress an excess of that you're treating it terribly. You will stress you're treating it terribly. That is OK, we as a whole do. You're not treating it terribly. There's no ideal method to do it, simply be cheerful you're doing it.

Try not to stress over clearing the psyche. Heaps of individuals ponder clearing your psyche, or halting all contemplations. It's most certainly not. This can now and then occur, yet it's not the "objective" of reflection. On the off chance that you have considerations, that is ordinary. We as a whole do. Our cerebrums are thought production lines, and we can't simply close them down. Rather, simply attempt to work on concentrating, and practice some more when your brain meanders.

Remain with whatever emerges. At the point when contemplations or emotions emerge, and they will, you may take a stab at remaining with them for some time. Indeed, I realize I said to come back to the breath, yet after you practice that for seven days, you may likewise have a go at remaining with an idea or feeling that emerges. We will in general need to maintain a strategic distance from emotions like dissatisfaction, outrage, uneasiness … however an incredibly valuable contemplation practice is to remain with the inclination for a little while. Simply remain, and be interested.

Become more acquainted with yourself. This training isn't just about concentrating; it's tied in with figuring out how your brain functions. What's happening inside there? It's dim, yet by watching your brain meander, get baffled, maintain a strategic distance from troublesome emotions … you can begin to get yourself. Become companions with yourself. As you become more acquainted with yourself, do it with a well-disposed demeanor rather than one of analysis. You're becoming more acquainted with a companion. Grin and give yourself love.

Does a body examine? Something else you can do, when you become somewhat better at following your breath, is concentrate on each body part in turn. Start at the bottoms of your feet — how do those vibe? Gradually move to your toes, the highest points of your feet, your lower legs, right to the highest point of your head.

Notice the light, sounds, vitality. Somewhere else to put your consideration, once more, after you've practice with your breath for at any rate seven days, is the light surrounding you. Simply keep your eyes on one spot, and notice the light in the room you're in. One more day, simply center around seeing sounds. One more day, attempt to see the vitality in the room surrounding you (counting light and sounds). Truly submit yourself. Don't simply say, "Sure, I'll attempt this for two or three days." Really invest in this. In your psyche, be secured, for at any rate a month.

You can do it anyplace. In case you're voyaging or something comes up toward the beginning of the day, you can do reflection in your office. In the recreation center. During your drive. As you walk some place. Sitting contemplation is the best spot to begin, yet in truth, you're rehearsing for this sort of care in all your years.

Follow guided reflection. On the off chance that it encourages, you can have a go at following guided reflections to begin with. My significant other is utilizing Tara Brach's guided reflections, and she discovers them extremely accommodating.

Check in with companions. While I like reflecting alone, you can do it with your life partner or youngster or a companion. Or then again simply make a responsibility with a companion to check in each morning after contemplation. It may assist you with staying with it for more.

Discover a network. Surprisingly better, discover a network of individuals who are pondering and go along with them. This may be a Zen or Tibetan people group close to you (for instance), where you proceed to ruminate with them. Or on the other hand locate an online gathering and check in with them and pose inquiries, get support, energize others. My Sea Change Program has a network that way.

Grin when you're set. At the point when you're done with your two minutes, grin. Be appreciative that you had this uninterrupted alone time, that you stayed with your responsibility, that you gave yourself that you're dependable, where you set aside the effort to become more acquainted with yourself and warm up to yourself. That is a stunning two minutes of your life.

CHAPTER 5

30 DAY CHALLANGE TO END EMOTIONAL EATING

This is an enthusiastic eating diary multi day challenge that is explicitly intended to assist you with halting your passionate eating, quit feeling remorseful or embarrassed about your eating, and discover your way to a cheerful and copious spot.

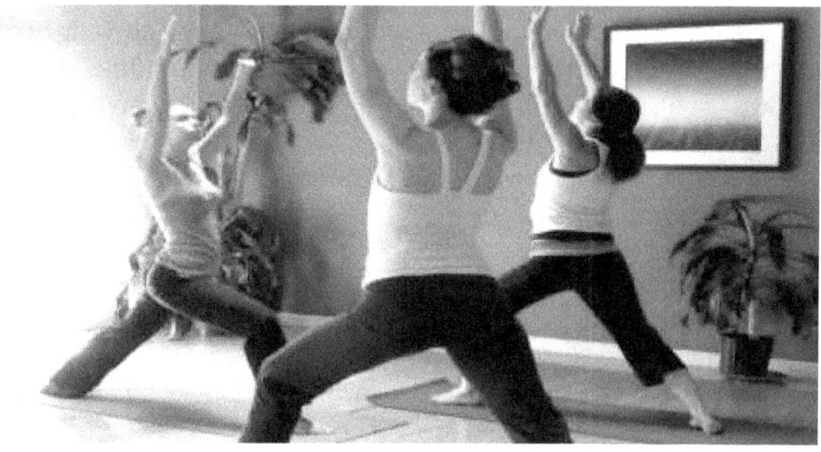

They're so much enjoyment, it's such a possible time period, and you get such a sentiment of achievement. What's not to cherish?

Despite the fact that the entire 'accomplish something for 30 days and it'll turn into a propensity' thing is a fantasy, it sure doesn't hurt. In case you're hoping to make something a piece of your life, doing a multi day challenge is a cool method to make a beginning.

What's more, in the event that you haven't took a stab at journaling, presently your possibility.

Attempt this wonderful enthusiastic eating diary multi day challenge that is explicitly intended to assist you with breaking the cycle and eat glad!

- **For What Reason Do A Passionate Eating Diary?**

You can get familiar with a ton and make your body, self, and life better. Sounds extraordinary right?

Journaling isn't just incredible enjoyment and a superb learning device, it is very brave mending benefits as well. As this brilliant article from the American Psychological Association diagrams, numerous individuals in some entirely awful circumstances can profit extraordinarily from journaling about their anxieties and battles. The exploration condensed in the article brings up that it doesn't generally make a difference what your identity is, or how or where you compose, yet that the demonstration of composing reflecting-and learning can be very advantageous, both truly and mentally.

They do pressure that it's the learning and reflecting piece of the journaling procedure that is vital. You can't simply expound on what you did today, close up your diary, and anticipate that the advantages should come in. You need to discover significance and development in your composition. How you compose your story and discover the implications in it will bigly affect your results.

- **In what capacity can a passionate eating diary help you?**

On the off chance that you've been living with, working with, or recuperating enthusiastic eating for whenever by any means, I'm certain you're very much aware that it's about far beyond just nourishment or eating. Truth be told, for a great many people, it's scarcely about those things by any stretch of the imagination. Enthusiastic eating is a message, an indication, and something to be investigated. Journaling is a phenomenal method to do a portion of this investigation.

As I've said over, the aftereffects of your journaling will truly rely upon how you compose your story and discover implications in yourself. This has immense potential for enthusiastic eaters! On the off chance that your enthusiastic eating has implications and messages, investigating them through composing can give bits of knowledge and development you'd never thought of.

You burrow inside yourself to put words to feelings and encounters, you can see associations occurring on the page, and your brain can open up to investigate regions that are new, or find new associations and implications in regions you've been over a million times inside your own head.

When you have a more profound comprehension of what's happening, you are in such a more grounded position to mend your passionate eating from the main drivers rather than yet another bandage convenient solution.

Guided Meditation To Help You Control Hunger And Release Stress

At the point when you consider weight reduction, your brain may quickly go to abstain from food and exercise. Be that as it may, investigate recommends care can assume a key job in overseeing desires, boosting mental self view, and cultivating good dieting and exercise propensities. It bodes well. Slow down to inhale, check out your body's sensations and feelings, and distinguish genuine appetite signals. These are for the most part methodologies that urge individuals to be completely present while getting a charge out of nourishment. Our specialists clarify four different ways you can utilize contemplation for weight reduction and its advantages.

- **You Become Increasingly Mindful Of Your Dietary Patterns.**

"Reflection is an extraordinary method to assist you with getting mindful of and associated with your considerations and activities," says Dr. Candice Seti, a clinical analyst, guaranteed fitness coach, and nourishment mentor who works with customers on way of life changes for weight reduction and support. "This is particularly gainful with regards to eating practices.

A great deal of us eats rapidly or without consideration. We don't genuinely acknowledge or make the most of our nourishment, nor do we value our craving or satiation levels. Careful reflection during eating times can help moderate our eating. [It] permits us to concentrate on how we are feeling during our dinners. After some time, this can assist us with figuring out how to recognize signs of satiation. So we quit eating when we are full instead of when our plate is vacant. It makes eating a cognizant conduct as opposed to a drive and can eventually quit indulging and pigging out."

As indicated by Joy Rains, creator of Meditation Illuminated: Simple Ways to Manage Your Busy Mind, you can utilize reflection to create attention to how and what you eat. She recommends seeing things, for example, the smell and temperature of the nourishment you're going to eat, your mood, your eating pace, and the size of each nibble.

"These exercises are segments of reflection. Putting your fork down between nibbles to permit time to give your body signs of totality," says Tania Elliott, M.D., boss clinical official at EHE. "Consider each chomp you take. How it smells, looks, tastes, and feels in your mouth, on your tongue, and between your teeth. This is a type of guided contemplation and care. [It] causes focus your attention to the nourishment you are eating as opposed to scarfing down your nourishment to attempt to 'treat' your on edge or tragic sentiments."

David Greuner, M.D., head specialist at NYC Surgical Associates, noticed that reflection is a viable technique to control pressure and improve mind-body availability. While contemplation doesn't ensure weight reduction, includes clinical clinician Alexis Conason, Psy.D., a lot of research backs up the medical advantages of reflection, especially around feelings of anxiety and generally speaking prosperity. Dietitian Kelsey Kinney recommends contemplation for weight reduction since it can improve your gut wellbeing and diminish aggravation.

- **Hoping To Get More Fit? Look At Aaptiv's Health Improvement Plan.**

This association with stress and uneasiness is twofold, Seti says. It's identified with both passionate eating and the arrival of specific hormones. "Individuals under incessant pressure regularly wind up utilizing nourishment as a way of dealing with stress. Indulging or weight gain is a characteristic outcome," she says. "Contemplation is an extraordinary method to control your feelings of anxiety, so comfort eating gets pointless. At the point when you are focused on, your body discharges cortisol to manage it. So your craving increments and your body begins putting away more midsection fat, the two of which seriously upset weight reduction endeavors. Reflection discharges oxytocin and serotonin, which check the impacts."

- **It Empowers More Advantageous Nourishment Choices.**

Stress eating is typical, to a degree. We as a whole know the sentiment of getting a charge out of a cupcake in the wake of a difficult day. In any case, there's a major contrast between eating your feelings and eating since you're really ravenous. Nourishment and emotional wellness go inseparably, Elliott says. Individuals frequently eat when they are pushed, exhausted, pitiful, or discouraged. Reflection methods, for example, single-entrusting or remaining present, assist you with diverting in those minutes. They can even diminish voraciously consuming food and passionate eating.

"Be available to what you're placing into your body," says Joe Burton, originator and CEO of While, an advanced prosperity preparing stage for representatives. "As opposed to that routine burger or pizza, you can prepare yourself to settle on better nourishment choices. Such a large number of us snatch a speedy dinner, or more terrible, inexpensive food, and go through a short lunch. As a matter of fact easing back down, settling on solid decisions and afterward eating your supper gradually as opposed to wolfing it down has huge advantages. Easing back down during dinners causes the cerebrum to recoup from consistently on mode. In any case, it likewise perceives when you're full. At the point when the brain is available, it's simpler to stay away from that subsequent making a difference."

- **Reflection Can Bolster Your General Weight Reduction Objectives.**

"Contemplation offers you the chance to profoundly consider all features of why you indulge, why you maintain a strategic distance from exercises, or whatever other issues that cause you to feel like you have to get in shape," Greuner says. "When considering this in a tranquil, [un]stressed condition, you can decide an answer and modify your propensities toward a more advantageous way of life."

Day by day contemplation can improve your relationship with nourishment, body, development, and the sky is the limit from there, Conason says. Utilizing representation methodologies, for example, envisioning your weight reduction objective or envisioning yourself partaking in practices that help your wellbeing objectives, can help with inspiration. "Reflection surely doesn't give any sort of enchantment in making weight reduction," Seti notes. "Yet, it can significantly affect certain parts of our wellbeing and eating that do majorly affect weight reduction."

CHAPTER 6

WHAT IS MEANT BY DIET

Does "diet" promptly make you think about a disagreeable weight reduction routine?

In the event that it did, you are presumably not the only one. For instance, consider the utilization of the expression "diet" in advertising nourishment items—it as a rule depicts food sources low in calories, for example, diet pop.

Be that as it may, there is another importance of this word. Diet can likewise allude to the nourishment and drink an individual devours every day and the psychological and physical conditions associated with eating. Sustenance includes more than essentially eating a "decent" diet—it is about sustenance on each level. It includes associations with family, companions, nature (the earth), our bodies, our locale, and the world.

Decisions about sustenance are especially connected to other people and other life shapes on this planet, so solid (and unfortunate) choices have extraordinary effect.

- **How many types of diet are there? And all work but is the mind that makes a different**

Consider it. Your mind is consistently "on." It deals with your musings and developments, your breathing and heartbeat, your faculties — it buckles down all day, every day, even while you're snoozing. This implies your mind requires a steady stockpile of fuel. That "fuel" originates from the nourishments you eat — and what's in that fuel has a significant effect. Set forth plainly, what you eat straightforwardly influences the structure and capacity of your mind and, at last, your state of mind.

Like a costly vehicle, your cerebrum capacities best when it gets just premium fuel. Eating great nourishments that contain loads of nutrients, minerals, and cancer prevention agents feeds the mind and shields it from oxidative pressure — the "squander" (free radicals) delivered when the body utilizes oxygen, which can harm cells.

Tragically, much the same as a costly vehicle, your mind can be harmed in the event that you ingest something besides premium fuel. In the event that substances from "low-premium" fuel, (for example, what you get from handled or refined nourishments) get to the cerebrum, it has little capacity to dispose of them. Diets high in refined sugars, for instance, are destructive to the mind. Notwithstanding declining your body's guideline of insulin, they additionally advance aggravation and oxidative pressure. Various examinations have discovered a connection between's an eating regimen high in refined sugars and weakened mind work — and even a compounding of side effects of disposition issue, for example, wretchedness.

It bodes well. In the event that your mind is denied of acceptable quality nourishment, or if free radicals or harming incendiary cells are coursing inside the cerebrums encased space, further adding to mind tissue injury, results are normal. Interesting that for a long time, the clinical field didn't completely recognize the association among state of mind and nourishment.

Today, luckily, the expanding field of nourishing psychiatry is discovering there are numerous results and relationships between's not just what you eat, how you feel, and how you at last act, yet additionally the sorts of microorganisms that live in your gut.

- **How The Nourishments You Eat Influence How You Feel**

Serotonin is a synapse that manages rest and craving, intervene states of mind, and hinder torment. Since about 95% of your serotonin is created in your gastrointestinal tract, and your gastrointestinal tract is fixed with a hundred million nerve cells, or neurons, it bodes well that the internal activities of your stomach related framework don't simply assist you with processing nourishment, yet additionally direct your feelings. Furthermore, the capacity of these neurons — and the creation of synapses like serotonin — is exceptionally affected by the billions of "good" microscopic organisms that make up your intestinal microbiome. These microscopic organisms assume a fundamental job in your wellbeing.

They secure the coating of your digestion tracts and guarantee they give a solid obstruction against poisons and "awful" microscopic organisms; they limit irritation; they improve how well you retain supplements from your nourishment; and they enact neural pathways that movement straightforwardly between the gut and the mind.

Studies have thought about "customary" eats less carbs, similar to the Mediterranean eating routine and the conventional Japanese eating routine, to a normal "Western" eat less carbs and have demonstrated that the danger of misery is 25% to 35% lower in the individuals who eat a conventional eating regimen. Researchers represent this distinction in light of the fact that these conventional eating regimens will in general be high in vegetables, organic products, natural grains, and fish and fish, and to contain just humble measures of lean meats and dairy. They are likewise drained of prepared and refined nourishments and sugars, which are staples of the "Western" dietary example. What's more, huge numbers of these natural nourishments are matured, and consequently go about as common probiotics.

This may sound unlikely to you, yet the thought that great microbes not just impact what your gut processes and assimilates, yet that they likewise influence the level of aggravation all through your body, just as your state of mind and vitality level, is picking up footing among scientists.

- **Nourishing Psychiatry: What Does It Mean For You?**

Begin focusing on how eating various nourishments causes you to feel — at the time, yet the following day. Have a go at eating a "perfect" diet for a little while — that implies removing every single prepared nourishment and sugar. Perceive how you feel. At that point gradually bring nourishments once again into your eating routine, individually, and perceive how you feel.

At the point when a few people "go clean," they can't accept how much better they feel both truly and inwardly, and how much more terrible they at that point feel when they reintroduce the nourishments that are known to upgrade aggravation.

Meditation For The Weight Watcher

Can you truly ruminate in a couple taken minutes? Of course, says Suze Yalof Schwartz, CEO and originator of Unplug Meditation. "At whatever point you can press it in and for whatever measure of time, that is acceptable," Schwartz says.

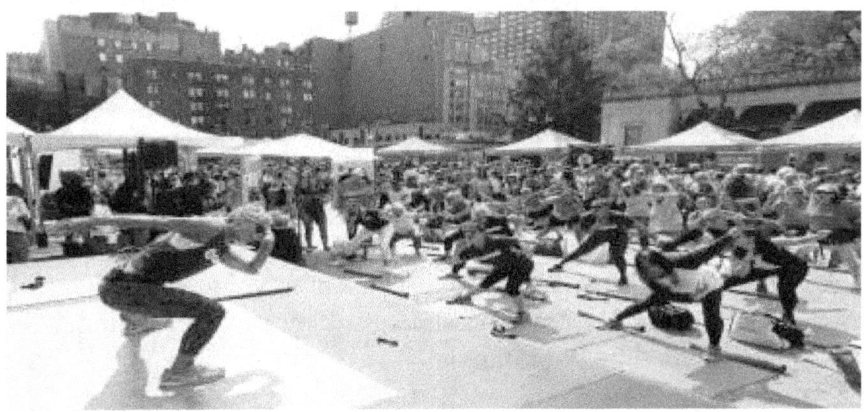

Indeed, a brisk meeting may be best, particularly in case you're different to it. "Your psyche's going to continually meander, and it'll be a fight among thought and center," Schwartz says. Finding the hole between the two, she says, is the sweet spot, and it gets simpler the more frequently you do it.

Similarly that a particular length of contemplation time isn't required, Schwartz says you don't have to sit a specific way or feel constrained to purchase props like reflection explicit cushions or candles. To put it plainly, contemplation ought not add more worry to your life. "It should meet you where you are," she says. "It's extremely simply relaxing."

One thing you do require, nonetheless, is where you won't be upset or disturbed. Schwartz says she's been known to bolt her vehicle entryways and ponder in a parking garage. "You will never discover an opportunity to ponder," she says. "You truly need to make it and cut it out of your day. Regardless of whether that is 60 seconds every day or an hour daily, it's all acceptable." For your next fast meeting, attempt one of these reflections from her book, Unplug: A Simple Guide to Meditation for Busy Skeptics and Modern Soul Seekers.

On the off chance that you have 1 moment to ponder, attempt …

❖   **THE SAVORING MEDITATION**

This is extraordinary for easing back down, valuing the occasion, advancing careful eating, and encountering what Schwartz calls "nourishment euphoria." Do it as you start a feast or tidbit.

❖   **GRASP THE NOURISHMENT.**

Take a gander at it and ask yourself, "How did this get from the earth to my fingers?" Think about it. Envision all the means it took to make a trip right to you. Lift the nourishment to your ear. At the point when you crush a few nourishments, they make intriguing sounds. Put in no time flat tuning in.

Put the nourishment before your mouth with your lips shut. Notice that you're salivating a little in expectation. Spot it in your mouth and feel the surface with your tongue, at that point start to bite as gradually as you can, seeing the same number of components as you can. Swallow, grin, and go on with your day.

In the event that you have 5 minutes to ruminate, attempt …

❖   **A QUICK SHOT OF CALM**

Perfect for easing uneasiness, chilling annoyance, or discharging dissatisfaction, this is the contemplation to go to when pressure is running high or in case you're going to talk freely or settle on an intense choice.

Take seven moderate breaths, breathing in and breathing out through your nose.

Take seven all the more moderate breaths, breathing in through your nose and breathing out through your mouth. At last, take seven all the more moderate breaths, breathing in and breathing out through your mouth. Resume breathing ordinarily and notice how your vitality has moved.

CHAPTER 7

FAST SAFE WEIGHT LOSS UNLOCKED

There are the best strategies for quick safe loss of weight than hardship, do you think about them? The greater part of Americans is gigantic or beefy. Nearness of the huge nourishment plan is last premise, yet one of things number one from which there are a great deal of endeavors of the individuals, keeping to an eating regimen with certain degrees of hardship as opposed to examining the best fat consuming rundown of acknowledgment to start.

I talk as a matter of fact. I know, since I was one of those individuals. I have begun to battle with my weight when I was in the lesser exceptionally.

Additionally what happens when you begin to jingle over once more? All things considered, you, most perhaps, become significantly huger, than you were, previously, on the grounds that your body has diminished now and the balanced muscles which you have lost, supplanting now with fat.

Frequently result is the thing that you reestablish a cycle over and over. I was there. It isn't charming and on the off chance that you were on this spoiled wheel of a hamster, than I trust these helps which worked for my companion considerably after nearness of three young people, without investing me being more straightforward.

Here Is Some Data, Which You Can Use To Arrive At Quick Safe Loss Of Weight: Food is something that can be convoluted. I can't let you know, what number of articles, books, painstakingly explored workshops and tuned in regarding a matter of quick safe loss of weight.

Fundamentally, when nourishment territories switch their cognizance of what is lovely for you and what isn't, it leaves you blended. You can wish to do buys in the business sectors of ranchers for most of your meat and to make for crude, new staple. It will independently hold you from the prepared staple.

Presently, you, most likely, have considered it before on the grounds that I have heard it from every dietician and the fitness coach with whom I have reached. Bite on 5-6 littler nourishment on all degree of day, rather than 3 major nourishments, and keep away from it inside four hours after your season of a fantasy. The supper before that can hit the sack to screw your fantasy. In certain individuals, it causes indigestion in light of the fact that the body eases back down around evening time.

It is safe to say that you are actually a peruser of a mark? We should put it in troublesome terms. Here is somewhat prophetic, offered by specialists of general wellbeing administrations. Maintaining a strategic distance from what you eat: the sugar, the advanced flour, the satisfied fats, high syrup of grain of fructose and oil.

You can be astonished to discover that something can hinder your framework which meddles with you to arrive at weight misfortunes. High syrup of grain of fructose is one of hoodlums who causes it. A considerable lot of you have appalled to prepare, however here is a little tip, I have gotten news from the individual master who says that most of individuals don't want particularly to be on the acknowledgment program.

On the off chance that you need some assistance to get thinner quick – you should toward the start comprehend that weight reduction isn't a fantasy. You do can shed pounds quick, this is conceivable, if you know the mysteries of weight reduction industry and its items.

How To Choose A Meditation

Regardless of appearances, the demonstration of contemplation is more than basically sitting peacefully for a while. It is the start of an excursion into the internal profundities of your heart and brain. It is through the investigation of these profundities where we tap into our actual wants and build up a comprehension of what our identity is and what one of a kind abilities and endowments we can bring to the world. However, sooner or later in one's reflection venture we may pose the inquiry, "What contemplation style is truly best for me?"

Reflection can possibly offer some wondrous advantages, yet it tends to be overpowering to pick a style. On account of its notoriety, there are numerous choices to browse and the web has a great deal to state about the subject. In case you're interested, the best activity is to begin attempting various ones. You will see a few people are alright with one contemplation style and others like to explore different avenues regarding various ones, and that is splendidly fine. It's imperative to discover one that suits you and supports where you're at throughout everyday life.

The Gifts of Meditation

As people, we are in steady motion, as is everything around us. Like the recurring pattern of sea tides, you may experience periods where you may need to make a few acclimations to get once again into "the stream" of your own cadence. Perhaps the best endowment of contemplation is figuring out how to be adaptable, and this turns out to be particularly significant with regards to your reflection practice. Picking a contemplation style ought to be peaceful; however it very well may be disheartening on the off chance that you aren't feeling the outcomes you are anticipating. Another significant exercise of contemplation is the idea of relinquishing desires.

There isn't a reflection that works superior to another. They all offer their own special advantages and every individual's experience differs also. Contingent upon what's happening throughout everyday life, here and there you may require more direction to help center or possibly you simply need to feel more joyful. It's useful to start seeing your rhythms and how you are getting along intellectually, truly, and profoundly, and afterward making modifications. These changes can be as large as leaving a place of employment that is unfulfilling or as little as saying thank you all the more regularly. Contemplation encourages you to realize what it is you have to do to enhance your life.

Reflection Self-Assessment

To start with, it's essential to initially registration with yourself and do a brisk appraisal. Don't hesitate to write down your reactions.

What do you feel is inadequate in your life?

•   How does your body feel? Are there any spots where it feels overwhelming or stuck?

•   Do you have a ton at the forefront of your thoughts, more than expected?

•   Do you need assistance centering?

How would you like to feel? Fed, associated, stimulated, intentional, and so on.

Try not to confine yourself to these inquiries. In the event that something different continues ringing a bell, pay heed to it. Your reactions to these inquiries will be useful in figuring out which style of reflection you may jump at the chance to attempt. Utilize this just as a guide and recollect that you will get profits by each reflection, maybe in some sudden ways. Contemplation is consistently there for you in the manner you need it to be. How about we investigate some reflection styles and check whether there is one that you may jump at the chance to attempt!

❖   GUIDED MEDITATION

Guided reflections are extraordinary for when you might want to be driven through an encounter. These should be possible by heading off to an in-person class, tuning in to an account, or adhering to any sort of verbal guidance. This style here and there requires some creative mind that comes normal to certain individuals. In case you're not one of those individuals, simply give a valiant effort and play "imagine." You will even now get a similar advantage. The subject or topic of the guided contemplation can be identified with physical prosperity, showing, plenitude, and so on.

- Helps learners who need some additional direction

- Helps dynamic personalities that need some assistance centering

- Assists with picking up clearness on territories of "stuckness"

There is a bounty of guided contemplations on the web. To assist you with beginning, attempt these guided reflections. PSM Online promotion

❖ **ADORING KINDNESS MEDITATION**

On the off chance that you need to begin changing your impression of the world, Loving-Kindness Meditation can start to help make this move. It utilizes words, pictures, and sentiments, to summon characteristics of adoration and cordiality toward yourself as well as other people. As of late, look into on this specific sort of contemplation has indicated a scope of advantages from improving general prosperity to giving alleviation from ailment and expanding social connectedness.

Advantages:

- Expands self esteem

- Improves associations with others

- Expands social associations

- Helps with physical mending

- Improves mental prosperity

You will discover a ton of incredible data on the web with respect to this point. This sound clasp is a genuine case of a Loving-Kindness Meditation.

❖ **CARE MEDITATION**

Contemplation envelops a wide scope of works on, including eating, strolling, watching the world, and even the more commonplace technique for sitting in stillness. Care is one such reflection practice that can be extraordinary. With its underlying foundations saturated with the Buddhist convention, care is a continuous life practice that encourages you to acknowledge all that emerges without judgment. It tends to what is happening at the time and attempts to discharge it immediately. You develop the act of giving up and setting consideration on that which causes you develop and advance a positive way. In the expressions of otherworldly pioneer and Buddhist priest, Thich Nhat Hanh: "Care causes you to return home to the present. What's more, every time you go there and perceive a state of satisfaction that you have, bliss comes."

Advantages

- Assists with pulling together consideration

- Diminishes pressure reaction

- Helps move toward a positive state of mind

- Improves mindfulness

- Improves wellbeing and prosperity

There are numerous approaches to rehearse care, including simply taking minutes for the duration of the day to see how you feel and what's happening around you. To assist you with beginning, this speedy contemplation method called "S.T.OP." can assist you with managing upsetting minutes. It permits you to stop, take in what's going on, and afterward act with more mindfulness and insight.

- Stop what you're doing.

- Slowly inhale and delay.

See what's going on in your psyche, body, and outer condition. Notice any default practices, for example, outrage, dread, and so on.

❖ **MANTRA MEDITATION**

This is a typical and darling reflection practice that will in general be progressively organized. "Mantra" signifies vehicle or instrument of the mind and can be utilized in various manners. Mantras can be sounds, words, or expresses and are regularly quietly rehashed for the span of a reflection, helping keep the brain centered and filling in as a vehicle to arrive at higher conditions of awareness. A few mantras are intended to have significance and others are utilized for their sounds or vibrations and deliberately have no importance.

Advantages

- Fulfills a requirement for structure

- Centers the meandering brain

- Diminishes pressure

- Improves mental and physical wellbeing

- Assists with picking up lucidity into your actual wants

When you begin investigating mantras, you will find that there are numerous accessible. Mantra reflection is best gained from a certified instructor, for example, those ensured through the Chopra Center where Primordial Sound Meditation is educated. You can likewise do a quest for instructors in your general vicinity. There are various strategies accessible to learn; don't hesitate to attempt them all or stick to whichever one you appreciate rehearsing.

❖   **RELAXING**

You may will in general invest a ton of energy pondering the past or the future while overlooking the most significant minute: "the now" or "the present." You don't have command over changing the past or future, yet you do have power over the present. What you do today influences tomorrow.

The act of a breathing reflection can assist you with bringing your concentration once more into the current minute so you can settle on progressively cognizant choices. The advantages are regularly felt promptly as the brain body association gets built up. As the brain quiets, so does the body and the other way around. A breathing reflection or practice can assist you with understanding and acknowledge how you can impact your own physical and mental prosperity.

Advantages

- Decreases pressure right away

- Assists with establishing

- Clears and focuses the psyche

- Revives the body

- Improves physical prosperity

You can take in increasingly about breathing procedures from yoga studios or wellbeing focuses in your general vicinity. Additionally, the web gives a lot of instructional exercises.

A breathing practice that can be very quieting is called Nadi Shodhana. You can play out this anyplace and whenever you start to feel some pressure. By and large, it's useful to begin with a breathing practice before going into your normal contemplation.

Utilize this as a manual for assist you with picking a style of reflection you may get a kick out of the chance to attempt. There are numerous parts of contemplation styles out there, however the couple of referenced here are acceptable passages into investigating this significant day by day practice. Keep it straightforward and play around with this procedure! You will know when you have discovered a style that impacts you.

CHAPTER 8

MEDITATION AND BREATHING - SUGGESTIONS FOR BEGINNERS

Contemplation is a way to deal with preparing the brain, like how wellness is a way to deal with preparing the body. Be that as it may, numerous contemplation methods exist — so how would you figure out how to ruminate?

"In Buddhist custom, the word 'contemplation' is proportional to a word like 'sports' in the U.S. It's a group of exercises, not a solitary thing," University of Wisconsin neuroscience lab executive Richard J. Davidson, Ph.D., revealed to The New York Times. What's more, unique reflection rehearses require distinctive mental abilities.

It's very hard for an apprentice to sit for a considerable length of time and consider nothing or have a "vacant psyche." We have a few devices, for example, an amateur reflection DVD or a cerebrum detecting headband to help you through this procedure when you are beginning. When all is said in done, the simplest method to start pondering is by concentrating on the breath — a case of one of the most widely recognized ways to deal with reflection: fixation.

❖ **FIXATION CONTEMPLATION**

Fixation contemplation includes concentrating on a solitary point. This could involve following the breath, rehashing a solitary word or mantra, gazing at a light fire, tuning in to a monotonous gong, or tallying dots on a mala. Since centering the brain is testing, a novice may reflect for just a couple of moments and afterward work up to longer terms.

Right now reflection, you just pull together your mindfulness on the picked object of consideration each time you notice your psyche meandering. Instead of seeking after arbitrary musings, you essentially let them go. Through this procedure, your capacity to focus improves.

❖   CARE CONTEMPLATION

Care contemplation urges the professional to watch meandering musings as they float through the psyche. The expectation isn't to engage with the musings or to pass judgment on them, however essentially to know about each psychological note as it emerges.

Through care contemplation, you can perceive how your musings and sentiments will in general move specifically designs. After some time, you can turn out to be progressively mindful of the human propensity to rapidly pass judgment on an encounter as fortunate or unfortunate, charming or upsetting. With training, an inward equalization creates.

In certain schools of reflection, understudies practice a blend of focus and care. Numerous controls call for stillness — to a more noteworthy or lesser degree, contingent upon the instructor.

❖   OTHER CONTEMPLATION STRATEGIES

There are different other contemplation strategies. For instance, a day by day contemplation practice among Buddhist priests centers legitimately around the development of sympathy. This includes imagining negative occasions and reevaluating them in a positive light by changing them through empathy. There are likewise moving reflection methods, for example, judo, qigong, and strolling contemplation.

❖   ADVANTAGES OF REFLECTION

On the off chance that unwinding isn't the objective of reflection, it is regularly an outcome. During the 1970s, Herbert Benson, MD, a specialist at Harvard University Medical School, authored the expression "unwinding reaction" in the wake of directing exploration on individuals who rehearsed supernatural contemplation. The unwinding reaction, in Benson's words, is "an inverse, automatic reaction that causes a decrease in the action of the thoughtful sensory system."

From that point forward, concentrates on the unwinding reaction have recorded the accompanying transient advantages to the sensory system:

- Lower circulatory strain

- Improved blood dissemination

- Lower pulse

- Less sweat

- More slow respiratory rate

- Less nervousness

- Lower blood cortisol levels

- More sentiments of prosperity

- Less pressure

- More profound unwinding

Contemporary specialists are currently investigating whether a reliable reflection practice yields long haul benefits, and noticing constructive outcomes on cerebrum and safe capacity among meditators. However it merits rehashing that the motivation behind reflection isn't to accomplish benefits. To put it as an Eastern savant may state, the objective of reflection is no objective. It's essentially to be available.

In Buddhist way of thinking, a definitive advantage of reflection is freedom of the psyche from connection to things it can't control, for example, outside conditions or solid inner feelings. The freed or "illuminated" expert no longer unnecessarily follows wants or sticks to encounters, yet rather keeps up a quiet brain and feeling of internal concordance.

Instructions to think: Simple contemplation for learners

This reflection practice is a phenomenal prologue to contemplation procedures.

Sit or falsehood serenely. You may even need to put resources into a reflection seat or pad.

Close your eyes. We prescribe utilizing one of our Cooling Eye Masks or Restorative Eye Pillows if resting.

Put Forth No Attempt To Control The Breath; Just Inhale Normally

Concentrate on the breath and on how the body moves with every inward breath and exhalation. Notice the development of your body as you relax. Watch your chest, shoulders, rib confine, and gut. Essentially concentrate on your breath without controlling its pace or power. In the event that your psyche meanders, return your concentration back to your breath.

How to Overcome Obstacles That Keep Us from Meditating

Impediments are the open doors that have been put on your way to move you to move past your apparent constraints. Peruse how you can distinguish the kind of impediments you are as of now confronting, and how to conquer them.

❖   **REFLECTING AT THE SEA SHORE AT NIGHTFALL**

Let's be honest, obstructions are a piece of life and none of us have the playbook on the most proficient method to defeat them. As perfect as it might sound, evading obstructions is preposterous; despite the fact that you can figure out how to function with the vitality that makes them and defeat the thought that you are by one way or another at their leniency. Allows first recognize what obstructions are, the reason it's essential to beat them, and where they may entangle you.

❖   **DISTINGUISHING OBSTACLES**

A deterrent is whatever impedes you of accomplishing your objectives and carrying on with the existence you really want. Hindrances present themselves the minute you put your focus on something you need.

Consider this: Have you at any point been keen on somebody impractically and afterward you just surrendered without making your first move because of a paranoid fear of making a dolt of yourself? Shouldn't something be said about the zone of prosperity? Do you ever end up needing to settle on more advantageous nourishment decisions possibly to be wrecked when the server brings the treat menu highlighting a warm chocolate magma cake? Or on the other hand, perhaps you hit the rest button a couple of times such a large number of and you continue botching your window of chance for practicing before work. These are only a couple of the regular, everyday deterrents that can lose you follow and messed up.

Why beating is snags significant? Deterrents wreck you. They keep you stuck in the past by keeping you from making a move. They root you in dread, persuading you that you aren't adequate, you don't know enough, you need more time or cash and you're out of choices. In the event that you don't figure out how to defeat hindrances, you show the danger of being controlled to them.

As a rule, impediments are physical or conspicuously self-evident, though some are non-physical and less discernable. Somehow or another they can appear as constraining convictions you have about yourself or others, and on certain days they show up as others or conditions keeping you from being, doing, or having the things you need. Snags appear in numerous structures and are experienced all through the vigorous (profound), mental, passionate, and physical bodies.

❖   VIGOROUS OBSTACLES

Vigorous obstructions are things that give you the sentiment of being drained or depleted constantly. They appear as everyday decisions that you are making in your life that lead to a lopsidedness in vitality yield versus vitality input.

Investing 75 percent of your time working and leaving next to no vitality to put toward solid sustenance, work out, or down time will bring about laziness, lack of concern, or all out burnout. A significant number of us will in general give more than we get and eventually, the imbalance will incur significant damage.

Attempt The Accompanying Activity To Assist You With Conquering Fiery Snags:

Invest some energy taking a gander at the territories throughout your life where there is an absence of congruity. Make a rundown of the things you are doing that you are giving a lot of your time and vitality. Scribble down a surmised level of time you spend for each.

Take a gander at the everyday issues or things you do that give you more vitality and demonstrate an inexact level of time you spend doing these things.

Toward the end, see where you can limit things that detract from your vitality levels and increment things that give you more vitality.

❖   MENTAL OBSTACLES

Mental obstructions regularly rotate around an absence of objectives, inspiration, or core interest. On the off chance that you don't have an objective, you don't have any course. It's close to difficult to get to where you're going in the event that you have no clue where it is you need to be.

Another psychological impediment is nonattendance of inspiration. Inspiration requires a degree of energy so as to continue progress ahead toward the objective. On the off chance that there is no inspiration, mental impediments will appear as obstruction and reasons.

A failure to remain concentrated on the final product can be a colossal impediment. "Pursuing squirrels" in your psyche—another term for being effectively diverted—is a typical subject for some individuals as we experience a daily reality such that performing multiple tasks has gotten celebrated. At the point when you're dissipated and not ready to keep up your center, you begin to turn out and are effectively tossed into overpower.

❖   **PASSIONATE OBSTACLES**

Passionate obstructions appear most oftentimes as day by day stressors: aggravation toward others, constraining convictions about your own self-esteem, considerations around your powerlessness to achieve certain things, and negative feelings dependent on past encounters.

Not setting aside enough down effort to get present to—and experience—love, euphoria, appreciation, and bliss in your day by day life may leave you questionably feeling as if life itself is the obstruction.

Mental and passionate impediments are the place we will in general point the finger outward, accusing others or conditions for the status quo as opposed to assuming liability for our decisions.

❖   **PHYSICAL OBSTACLES**

Physical impediments will in general appear as an absence of time or cash, standards of conduct, and physiological reactions. For instance, in the event that you are somebody who battles with dealing with your time viably, you will experience issues completing things in an effective way—if by any means. In the event that you aren't in a budgetary section that underpins your requirements and objectives, this will appear as an undeniable test for you.

Unexpected disease and injury experienced in the physical body are snags that can incidentally lose you course. In case you're not speedy to mend—intellectually or truly—it might crash you for a considerable length of time or even years. In different cases, impediments may appear as social decisions like resting in light of the fact that you feel vivaciously, intellectually, or sincerely depleted.

❖ GUIDED MEDITATION FOR OVERCOMING OBSTACLES

Contingent upon how you manage the deterrents that current themselves will decide the recurrence and power of which you experience them. Following is a guided reflection for helping you to conquer obstructions in any part of your life. As you travel through every self-reflection question, permit yourself a moment or two for thought.

❖ SIT EASILY AND CLOSE YOUR EYES

Start to take moderate full breaths, in and out through your nose.

Permit your shoulders to unwind and your middle to mellow with each breathe out.

Bring into your mindfulness an aspect of your life where an impediment is available.

❖ CONSIDER WHEN, WHERE, AND HOW THIS IMPEDIMENT STARTED

Ask yourself who or what triggers the issue. What considerations and feelings are common when the hindrance is available?

Presently carry your consideration regarding the expense of this deterrent. How can it influence your capacity to be, do and have the things you need throughout everyday life? How can it influence everyone around you?

Next, see what can be accessible to you in the event that you conquer this deterrent and can move capably advance in your life.

Consider anybody you realize who has as of now conquered this sort of impediment. Who right? What approach did they take?

Presently consider how you may do things another way than the manner in which you have been so far, maybe including a few methodologies others have taken.

Next, welcome in a goal for an innovative answer for approach. Approach your Self or the Universe for direction in how best to explore and conquer this deterrent.

Furthermore, presently, envision your life as though the deterrent was broken up and you are currently remaining in the existence you have made by structure.

After you have a positive interior portrayal (a picture, sound, or sentiment) of being liberated from this obstruction, put in almost no time in calm consideration before gradually coming out of your reflection.

After coming out of your contemplation, you might need to write down any musings into a note pad or diary so you have some unmistakable subtleties to then transform into significant advances. It's imperative to adopt an empathetic strategy to this procedure and truly permit yourself to feel into your feelings, tuning in for your inward direction to deliver the understanding you need.

Keep in mind; hindrances are the open doors that have been put on your way to move you to move past your apparent impediments. Recognizing them is only the initial phase in making enduring change in your life. The finish and making a move to beat them is the place the genuine gold is.

CHAPTER 9

TIPS ON MEDITATING FOR A HEALTHY MIND AND BODY

❖   **DROP ALL WANTS AND ARRANGING**

The impediment for contemplation is the longing and all you're intending to accomplish something. Offer the craving through give up with the trust, "it is directly for me, it will be finished." Just figure it will occur and unwind. Give up implies the capacity to drop wants or botherations.

See the uselessness of the satisfaction of the craving and be without the heat of the longing. On the off chance that your craving doesn't get satisfied, it prompts dissatisfaction and causes wretchedness. Regardless of whether your wants get satisfied, so what? You are in a similar spot where nothing large has occurred. It has sat idle; it has not contacted you.

On the off chance that you want, want for the most noteworthy. At the point when you want truth, every other want drop off. You generally want something that isn't there however truth is consistently there. Want for truth evacuates every other want; at that point it will break up and what will remain is euphoria.

❖   **DEALING WITH VARIOUS FEELINGS**

During contemplation, in some cases you will encounter pity and different emotions may likewise come up yet they simply cruise by. Put your consideration more on the breath and on the sensations in the body. Each feeling has a relating sensation in the body and that sensation thusly makes that exact same feeling. An occasion made a feeling inside you and the feeling again makes a comparable sort of air around you and this cycle goes on. The best way to break the cycle is to watch the sensation as a sensation and de-interface it from feelings. It is basic. In the event that you think for only a short time, you will get that. It's clearer on an experiential level.

❖ BOREDOM IN REFLECTION

In the first place, reflection may be exhausting, yet this will change. Remain on. Go bit by bit. Contemplation is resting in yourself. Become the soothsayer from being the seen.

❖   UNDERSTAND THE TRANSIENT IDEA OF EMOTIONS

Try not to be your very own football sentiments. We are not captives of our feelings, yet we feel, 'Goodness! I feel like this', just as we are captives of our feelings. With center and assurance, you would not think much about the inclination.

The issue with sentiments is that we think emotions are the equivalent, steady. Emotions go back and forth, they change. You feel bravo time and afterward you feel awful, at that point you feel better and afterward you feel awful once more. On the off chance that you base your life on sentiments, at that point you will be no place.

Be submitted and resolve to accomplish something and do it. You realize the genuine fearlessness is to face your sentiments and not become your very own football emotions.

❖   QUIETEN THE PRATTLING MIND

Watch nature! At the point when you are watching, there is close association among watching and ingestion. Contemplation is ingestion. The initial step for reflection is watching. At the point when you are simply watching and watching, the babbling in the psyche gets lesser and lesser and it at long last vanishes it needs some expertise to stop this prattling mind.

On the off chance that you can't reflect in light of the fact that your brain is prattling, simply feel that you are a little dumb and afterward you would have the option to sink profound into contemplation.

Your mind is a little bit of the all out awareness. On the off chance that you are stuck in the insight, you miss a lot. Satisfaction is the point at which you rise above the keenness. In stunning or in feeling moronic, you rise above the insight

The Importance Of Food Education

If the body is provided with all nutrients, it becomes stronger. Lifespan not only increases but the quality of life also becomes better.

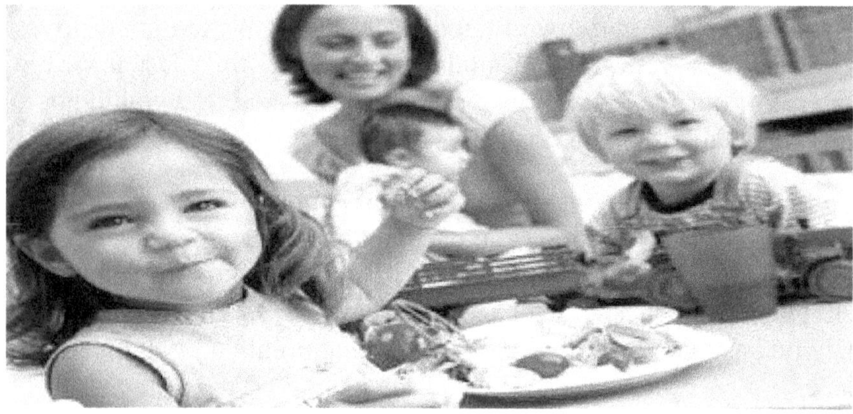

Understanding food encourages a good relationship with food. Food education is therefore important for both children and adults to betterment the quality of our lives.

Learning about food is important in influencing our behavior towards foods; if started at younger developing years, food education can promote good eating habits, good health and prevent diseases. This is achieved by the understanding of how immunity works, what deficiency causes low immunity and what can be done to increase immunity in the body.

It can also help in understanding deficiency diseases; understanding to consistently provide for the body what it needs to fight for itself and prevent the formation of hormones and cells that may encourage the development of deficiency diseases like diabetes and hypertension can go a long way in maintaining a healthier society.

Understanding food also encourages and promotes good mental health. In return, it promotes the eradication of food-related disorders such as obesity, anorexia, and bulimia which come about as a result of misunderstanding and misusing food to alter outward body appearance.

The functions of the brain are also strongly influenced by the kind of food we partake in. Understanding the **composites** of the brain and what we must or must not eat to maintain a healthy brain is fundamental for the functioning of the body and intelligent interactions. **Research Output**

People suffering from disability caused by mental illnesses are also on the rise. It is therefore important that every person learns about foods that promote the development and proper functioning of the brain while also strengthening the brain enough that it can fight off free radicals that damage the brain.

Not only does food education teach and inform us about disease preventive measures, but it also equips us with nutritional information that empowers us on how to maintain a healthy life. The balance of proteins, glucose, carbohydrates, fats, calcium, and water ensures that the body and mind are energized and functioning at maximum best.

We must understand the strong correlation between the food we consume and our character. The effects of food on character development can either promote or destroy wholeness. This extensively affects how we relate to food, with ourselves and with others. For example, people who suffer from food addiction, obesity, stress or depression also suffer from low self-esteem.

This means that they devalue their lives and hence they can easily cause harm on themselves by overindulging or denying themselves food. By feeling so bad about themselves, such patients tend to avoid other people. Development of character is, in this case, interfered with as there is no accountability or little to no human interaction.

By understanding food, we are also able to understand our physical being and understand why exercise is fundamental for our health. Food education helps us enjoy physical activity and promote community living.

Food education should be promoted worldwide, knowledge is after all power. Knowing what is important for your well being promotes and encourages a healthy eating culture. In the long run, it creates a healthy society that has adopted to good eating as a lifestyle.

CHAPTER 10

HOW TO STOP A DIET MENTALITY AND MAKE PEACE WITH FOOD

A person who loses weight through diet has a likelihood of regaining weight in less than a year. This is because dieting has a demanding effect on the body.

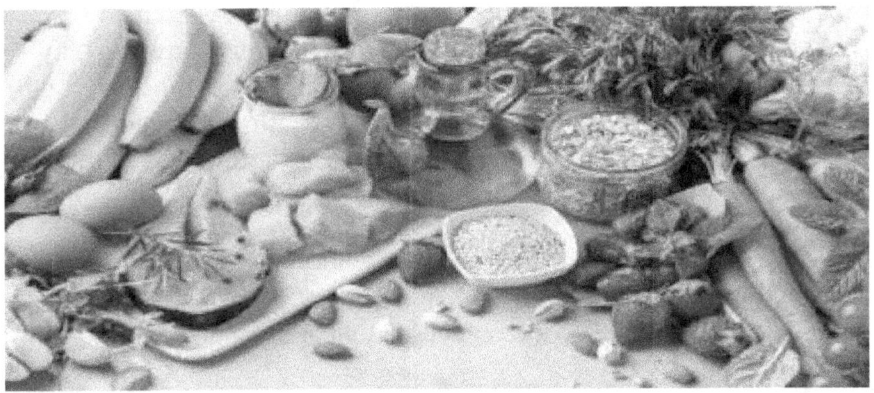

Dieting is the art of denying the body specific foods and creating a feeding schedule for the body to lose weight. Any time the body is denied food or introduced to a new regimen, the gut still remembers what it already knows. For this reason, the body will begin to behave as if it is being starved to death. The body will go into a 'defense' mechanism where it holds onto the fats in the body as a way of retaining its nutrients for longer periods. This results in cravings and binge eating because the body will register that it has been denied some food.

Instead of eating what the body needs, diet makes an individual stick to a rule or a habit that the body will work to fight against.

Restricting specific foods to your body will only make you want the food more. This is because the metabolism slows down and the hormones that regulate appetite change. Dieting is therefore not an advisable way of losing and maintaining favorable body weight.

Instead, people should adapt to a feeding friendly lifestyle. Every food is important for the body, however, potions and times of consumption is what should be observed while eating food. To have a proper eating lifestyle, we must understand how food works for our bodies. We must understand which foods provide the body with specific nutrients and understand a combination of foods that will nourish the body.

People must enjoy the foods that they eat. Taking time to savor the food chew and swallow will make digestion much easier and efficient for the body. Have a relationship with your body in a way that you can understand when the body tells you what it needs. It will soon become normal for you to understand what is important for you. However, if you do end up indulging in excessive carbs or artificial sugars, do not cause your body tension for eating when your body says it's not yet time.

Tension can lead to the release of stress hormones which will lead to cravings and eventually more unnecessary eating. Be kind on yourself.

What To Do When You Are Hungry

When you feel hungry, it is important that you feed your hunger with nutritious foods. Nutritionists' advice that we should have water and snacks in between meals to deal with hunger pangs. Staying hungry because of a diet plan will only make the body crave for more foods. Our bodies only crave sugar, carbohydrates, and fats which in excess are not good for health.

In the same spirit, a healthy lifestyle demands that we treat our bodies with respect. Overeating will only slow down metabolism, increase the accumulation of fats in the stomach and make digestion difficult for the body. We must realize when we have had enough. This we can only control when we consistently provide for our body with what it needs.

A healthier lifestyle gives a person more confidence than a diet which could leave persons questioning themselves or feeling hungrier. We must understand and internalize reasons as to why we eat so that we may have a good relationship with food without feeling the need to restrict our eating habits.

Understanding the effects of dieting is important to show you the need for an alternative feeding lifestyle. No one has come up with an ideal or perfect diet; the possibility of creating an eating disorder is greater to people who diet. This is because weight loss through dieting can change how the mind thinks; people may eat in small or large potions only to end up with eating disorders such as anorexia.

Learning The Art Of Dieting

Dieting has also created an illusion or perception that being tiny is being healthy, yet different people have different body to mass index (BMI). Whether big or small we must observe what is happening inside of our bodies that determine good health. Even though diabetes is common with people of bigger body frames, it is possible for small people who eat recklessly and to get the deficiency caused by disease. Hypertension is also common to people of all body types and sizes.

Dieting has caused a restriction in foods, a feeling that specific foods are good while others are bad. The truth of the matter is that all foods are good for the body. Understanding the potions and their needs in our systems is what is important. Eating a variety of foods is associated with good health.

The majority of the people who start on a diet plan can testify that diets are not a permanent way of life. The chances of the diet succeeding for the long term are close to none. This may affect individuals mentally because it leaves you with feelings of failure and despair. Eating disorders, malnutrition, and mental instability are born out of this.

CHAPTER 11

HOW TO ENSURE THE EATING DISORDER NEVER COMES BACK

When a person is experiencing an eating disorder there is an extreme disturbance of their eating habits. It is either they are not eating enough food for their body or they are eating more than they require. When they eat too little, the body lacks the necessary nutrients for it to function at its maximum best, when they eat too much the body is unable or struggles to process the food well enough. Fat deposits also increase in the body. All this leads to various eating disorders.

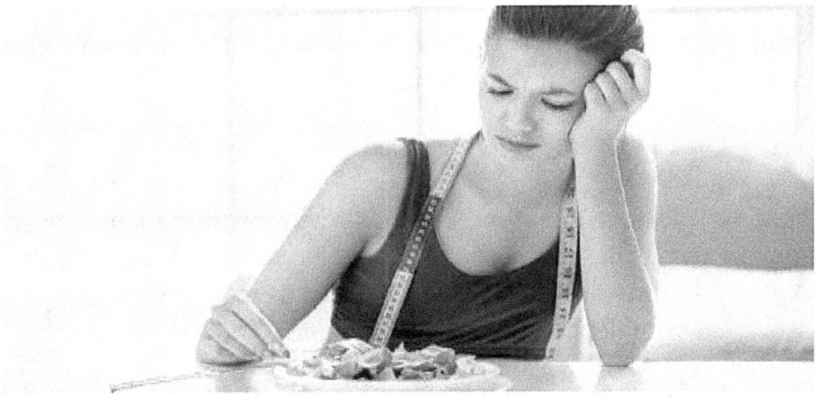

The root cause of these disorders is either eating too much food or eating too little food.

Restricting what a person eats is meant to give them control while overeating is to comfort and console someone's feelings.

Some of the **common eating disorders** that affect people

today are as described bellows;

❖   **ANOREXIA NERVOSA**

is an eating condition that affects people with low body weight. People who suffer from anorexia use unorthodox methods to prevent themselves from gaining weight. This could be by self-inducing unprescribed drugs and causing themselves to vomit so as not to gain weight. These people do anything to be thin. Their body to mass index is usually lower than that of an average human being of their age.

❖   **BULIMIA NERVOSA**

On the other hand, is a condition where a person eats a lot of food then immediately feels guilty and tries to get rid of the food? They can do this by causing themselves to vomit or ingesting laxatives.

❖   **BINGE EATING DISORDER**

People who suffer from binge eating uncontrollably consume large quantities of food over short periods.

❖   **OBESITY**

These people have knowingly or unknowingly accumulated large amounts of fats in their body, their body to mass index is usually above 30 Eating disorders are categorized as mental illnesses associated with depression and anxiety.

Eating disorders are known to cause serious illnesses and even death when the conditions are not managed in good time. People with this disorder are prone to heart attacks. Due to deficiency in nutrients and the accumulation of fats in the body, body organs are also prone to damage. Patients who suffer from this disorder must get psychological treatment

To treat and ensure that eating disorder never comes back, you have to find the underlying problem that causes a specific eating disorder.

There are environmental, psychological and biological factors that may cause eating disorders. Some of which can cause serious and chronic illnesses.

Some Of The Environmental Factors That May Cause Overeating Disorders Are;

Work; if you work in such a busy environment that you hardly find time to eat, you may eat on the go. This means that you do not have the chance to ensure that your meal has all the nutrients that your body requires. This also applies to travelers who end up eating more fast foods than organic foods.

Different cultural eating habits also cause an eating disorder. For example, some cultures advocate for drinking cold water or processed juices after a meal which only goes to slow metabolism and digestion.

Some Of The Biological Factors That May Cause Eating Disorder Are:

Genetic inheritance. When there is a history of overeating in the family it could be because of an appetite-inducing gene that is present and which can be passed from one generation to another.

Hormonal Imbalance Can Also Cause An Eating Disorder

Although it can be solved with proper meals, a lack of nutrients in the body is the leading cause of an eating disorder in the world.

Minimum self-respect People who look down on themselves tend to isolate themselves and find solace in food. This is likely to cause eating disorders.

People who are not confident in their bodies also have a high chance of eating disorders to make they feel good.

To ensure that eating disorder does not come back;

People must accept themselves and appreciate themselves as they are. Embracing your beauty in whatever form encourages confidence and high living standards.

When you accept yourself as you are, what others think or say about you becomes a non-issue. You also learn to take criticism and maintain an open mindset. This will interpret to better eating habits as you finally see that there is no need to match up with anything or anyone.

Build on your self-esteem by starting with how you look. Start by dressing smartly. When you look good, you feel good and have the desire to do things that make you feel even better about yourself. When you love yourself, your mental outlook on life changes and that greatly contributes to better eating habits.

Find better ways to deal with stress and anxiety as they come as they are the main reason people misuse food and end up with eating disorders. You can journal your daily activities as a way of coping with stress, take a hike or dance lessons, embark on music to help you elevate your mood without thinking about food.

Find and maintain good habits that will make your body and mind feel energized at all times.

A balanced diet, coupled up with exercising as a routine will result in good mental health thus avoiding eating disorders.

Make friends with food; understand your food intake concerning your body. Love food and know why you must eat different nutrients. People who have a good relationship with food hardly suffer from food-related disorders because they know how to manage their food intake according to their body needs at all times.

Ensuring that you get enough sleep will prevent insomnia (lack of sleep) which causes anxiety and stress throughout the day. As explained earlier, stress causes a release of hormones that cause cravings to the body. To prevent eating disorders, a person must have enough sleep every day. On average a person must sleep at least seven to eight hours a day.

Creating honest and good relationships with other people in your environment can play a big role in eradicating food-related disorders. People who suffer from food disorders often need encouragement to continue with good practices. Surrounding yourself with people who encourage your good habits and lovingly discourage your bad habits can push you towards healthy eating habits.

Anorexia and bulimia often lead to feelings of tiredness and irritability. This can be controlled if we eat balanced diets. Controlling the amount of proteins, carbohydrates, and sugar in your food can result in good feelings that will eradicate food disorder symptoms. Take a day at a time with good food and experience the relief that the body must feel.

Finally, patients suffering from eating disorders must seek the help of a physician and a psychiatrist for treatment. Talking to a trusted family member or friend is also a good place to begin finding help.

The Connection Between Mood And Food

As discussed in previous chapters, a high percentage of people use food to express their inner feelings. Sometimes they are positive feelings but at most times they are negative feelings.

It is easier to access fast foods when you are stressed or tired from work because they are readily available and affordable. When stress hormones are released from the body, body metabolism is lowered and more glucose is produced. This increases our energy levels and makes us more irritable.

The reason fast foods have always been the craving that feeds our feelings is because of the amount of carbohydrates found in the meals. When we feed on carbohydrates, the hormone serotonin is increased; this helps us deal with our hunger pangs and calms us down.

The relationship between our food and mood has become a symbiotic relationship. What you eat can affect your mood and vice Versa. For example, when you are stressed, stress hormones are released from the body; this derails your energy and causes you to have a craving for carbohydrates, sugars, and fats.

How you feel can also affect what you eat. When you are happy or sad and you overindulge in food it slows your metabolism making you feel tired, week and sometimes sleepy too.

In the same way, when you eat too much protein and glucose filled foods, the body produces energy and triggers feelings of happiness.

Stress can also cause a loss in appetite as a short term effect. When the body is under duress it produces adrenaline, a hormone that triggers the body to temporarily shut down any desire to eat food.

Stressed people not only overindulge in food but also sleepless and exercise less. They are more likely to take alcoholic drinks in comparison to people who are not stressed. In large portions, alcohol could be harmful to the body. The body in a hurry secrets digestive hormones to deal with the alcohol first as the liver struggles to de-toxicity the body from alcohol. This results in extreme hunger the calls for more and more eating. The beverage also helps in the production of glucose which increases energy levels and desire to unnecessarily eat more food. This may result in obesity and other food-related disorders.

Are You Hungry Or Stressed

While hunger is generated from the stomach, emotional hunger is generated from the brain. It is therefore important that we train our brain to deal with different situations that may cause a substantial

mood change. To do this, we must understand the difference between real hungers from a pang of emotional hunger.

• 	Feeling real hunger happens gradually and increases over time. Hunger generated from a mood often presents itself as a feeling, it is sudden and urgent.

• 	Once you are done eating when you are really hungry, your mind moves on to think of other things. In emotional eating, you can't stop thinking about the food, how it tastes, how it smells or even its texture in the mouth and also how you want to eat more.

• 	When you are hungry, you will eat whatever food is presented to you. Emotional hunger, on the other hand, is a craving, you seek to eat a specific meal, often salty, greasy or sugary

• 	You stop eating once your body feels full when you are really hungry. When you are emotional eating, you do not get enough of the food. As soon as you are done eating you feel the need to have some more

It is, however, possible to **inspire good habits in spite of any**

mood. This is by;

- Keeping a journal to document how you feel rather than eating

- Regularly exercising your body so that you are mentally able to handle stress

- Meditation will allow you to understand yourself better and have control of how you feel over different situations

- Have a strong social support system. This will encourage you to be considerate not only when you make food choices but also other life choices

- Having a regular eating schedule. Do not give your body a chance to feel hungry or distressed

- Eating mindfully not only allows you to enjoy a meal but makes the digestion process easier and efficient for your body.

CHAPTER 12

IS FOOD CONTROLLING YOUR LIFE

Eating especially when in a bad mood, usually releases a hormone that makes a person feel good about them. The hormone responsible for this is called dopamine.

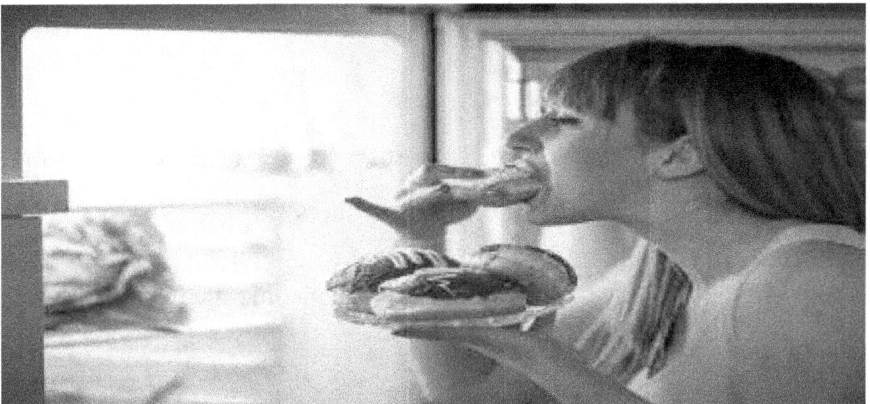

Production of dopamine in the body can have someone craving for this good feeling at all times. For this reason, it is possible that food can be addictive and control our lives.

Causes Of Food Addiction Are As Follows:

•   **Hormonal imbalance** is caused by a lack of nutrients in the body. Hormonal imbalance can cause low serotonin. This in result causes people, especially women to experience food cravings. This can easily grow to become a food addiction.

- Using specific medications can create a side effect of food addiction.

- Some people are genetically susceptible to food addition while others are exposed to foods high with artificial sweeteners, carbohydrates, and calories when they were still young.

- Victims of traumatic events like domestic violence or sexual violence can turn to eating comfort foods which then become an addiction

- People who are addicted to drugs also feel the need to consume large amounts of foods thus becoming addicts

- Grief or a loss of a loved one can push someone to find comfort in food thus birthing a food addiction.

- Abnormalities of the brain can also cause someone to be addicted to food as a way to feel good about themselves

- Food addiction can also be born out of bad eating habits.

As discussed in chapter six, there are ways to identify whether one is eating out of hunger or out of a mood. These same reasons will shade light or whether or not food is controlling your life.

For you to understand if food controls your life, you have to first understand food addiction.

This Is How You Identify Food Addiction:

• People addicted to food eat even when they are not hungry. They will eat because there is food on the table, a specific food smells good and because they are feeling happy or sad.

• Addicted people also eat more than what their body requires. Even when they feel full they continue to eat

• They eat unbelievably large portions of food and often hide some food to eat later when no one is looking.

• Food addicts are selfish with food. They will not want to share food even when they do not need it

• They also have regular food cravings; they crave foods that are filled with sugar, carbohydrates, and calories.

• People addicted to food experience a temporary feeling of relief after eating certain foods. Shortly after they are having fresh cravings and want more food.

Like any other addiction, food addiction also has its side effects. In some cases, food addiction has caused the rupturing of organs and even death.

Effects Of Food Depression

• Depression. Overeating can cause excessive production of hormones in the body. This results in low energy, weakness, and lack of motivation. All these lead to depression.

• Infertility issues. Women with higher body weight have a high chance of experiencing infertility problems. They also have a higher chance of suffering from diabetes and hypertension which can also affect their fertility

• Digestive issues. Overeating can cause bloating, constipation and diarrhea.

• Heart disease. Due to consuming large amounts of food, the level of cholesterol in the blood increases. This can lead to heart attack and heart failure.

• Isolation. Food addicts feel different from normal people. They are afraid of being judged, so they prefer to be alone most of the time.

• Obesity. As a result of overeating, the body accumulated fats causing a rise in the body to mass index and resulting in excessive body weight.

• **Self-esteem issues**. Due to the fear of being judged for being overweight or for poor eating habits, people with food addiction usually suffer from low self-esteem. They find themselves lacking confidence and feeling inadequate.

Even though it may require intervention, acceptance, diagnosis and psychological treatment, it is possible to **break away from food addiction**.

As an individual, you will need to;

•   Be aware of your food triggers. This could be salty food, artificial juices with artificial sweeteners or foods high in calories. Once you eat your trigger food, you end up craving for more and creating for yourself an eating disorder. It is therefore important that you know and keep away from your trigger.

•   Getting alternative self-care routine like a massage, taking a hike, meditation. Thus will keep you relaxed and steer your mind away from food.

•   Choose the right social circle or support group. The right group of people can identify your eating habits and call you out if they notice overeating. They can hold interventions and introduce n overeaters to overeaters anonymous to get assistance.

•   Eating regularly will also ensure that your body is nourished with all nutrients and therefore suppressing any unnecessary cravings.

How To Cope With Food Cravings

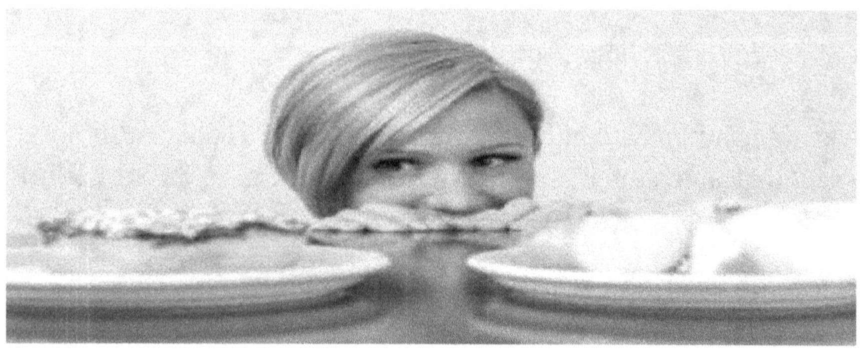

Food cravings originate from the brain and not the stomach as hunger does. For this reason, it is possible to control and manage our cravings. We must realize that every food is good for the body, however how and when we eat the food is what will influence the amount of nutrients we can sieve from it.

To cope with food cravings, we need to understand why we eat food in the first place.

The soul reason we consume food is to maximize the nutrients for survival. We eat to leave, so even in small potions, if we can provide the body with everything it needs, we can be able to leave healthy lives.

Understanding why we eat is important in creating a relationship with food and our body. This makes it easier for us to understand what our body needs. If the body receives all the nutrients it requires, the body will maintain the necessary balance and issues of hormone imbalance; mood and cravings will be unheard of. Understanding what we eat can also help us eliminate dieting as a short term solution to losing weight. Starving the body only regenerates cravings and causes even more consumption of food when the opportunity presents itself. Eating appropriate foods to balance sugar and provide energy for the body will prevent this from happening.

Planning meals to ensure that the body has everything it needs to function at all times will help to cab cravings. In one meal the body should be provided with enough vegetables, starch, and proteins. This will ensure that a person is full and that all nutrients have been given to the body.

Eating regularly and healthy snacking between meals will ensure that there is enough sugar balance in the body. This will prevent the secretion of hormones that cause cravings to happen.

Exercise To Lose Body Fat In The Mid-Body. More Fat In The Body Means More Cravings

Eating and drinking foods that catalyze the release of peptides, a hormone found in the gut that makes the stomach feel full will help curb cravings. Such foods include proteins and fiber.

Avoiding excess carbohydrates, calories and processed sugars also reduce cravings. These foods are referred to as trigger foods when you eat once, you will want more.

Do not stay idol, and the idol mind will crave for food. Destruct your mind from thinking about food.

Fight stress. Tension in the body will cause a release of stress hormones that cause cravings.

Water is a necessity for any living thing to survive; a person is likely to survive without food for a few days more than they are without water. Physician advice that a normal person must drink at list 2 liters of water in a day, this will keep the body hydrated, help with digestion and oxygen circulation in the body.

The majority of the times we feel hungry after having a filling meal, it's a sign that the body needs water. Before you feed your hunger, remember to drink water and the hunger feeling will go away.

It is also important that we consume warm water first thing when we wake up in the morning. This will keeps the body hydrated throughout the day and drives out toxins from the body.

Warm water causes several effects on our food habits and as a result of our cravings.

Benefits Of Water In Our Bodies.

•   Drinking warm water helps in digestion by opening up the stomach and allowing a smooth breakdown of foods.

•   It also fights cholesterol and obesity by breaking down fats and absorbing nutrients

•   Warm water also assists the body to get rid of harmful stomach acids and neutralizes the digestive juices.

•   It induces sleep by keeping the body warm and relaxed. How we sleep has a direct effect on our eating habits.

•   It regulates bowel movement

•   And also controls food cravings

Generally, warm water is essential for the body to function properly and for a healthy digestive system. This goes to ensure that the body keeps food cravings under control.

5 Ways To Strengthen Your Stress Resilience

❖   **YOGA SELF-CARE**

What makes a few of us ricochet back despite life's difficulties and others disintegrate? Why is it that, a few days, we feel ready to take on the world, while on different days, one seemingly insignificant detail can set us off? There are without a doubt various responses to these inquiries be that as it may, on a physiological level; analysts realize that our pressure strength levels are associated with a certain something: the emotional eating.

The emotional eating, our tenth cranial nerve, adjusts the parasympathetic sensory system, the piece of the sensory system that causes us to quiet down and unwind. Likewise called the "meandering nerve" since it wanders through the body, the emotional eating directs heart and breath rate and controls our voice tone, organs, and stomach related tract. From multiple points of view, the emotional eating is the air traffic controller of our physical body—sending and getting messages from the cerebrum about when to process, when to inhale, and what to feel. This makes it a fundamental player in building pressure versatility.

Strangely, the condition of our emotional eating can be estimated. Researchers built up a measure called pulse fluctuation, which tracks the time between hearts pulsates. When there is changeability between heart thumps, this suggests a high vagal tone, which is associated with great pressure flexibility. When there is little fluctuation between heart thumps, this suggests low vagal tone, which is related to poor pressure versatility. The primary concern? When there is adaptability in our pulses, as opposed to an inflexible beating, we are stronger. Sounds entirely like yoga, isn't that so? Adaptability implies versatility and improved general wellbeing.

Fortunately the emotional eating can be reinforced, through the way of life, practice, and aim. Here are a couple of practices that have been appeared to increment vagal tone.

❖   **SLOW, DEEP, BREATHING**

This training is without a doubt probably the most ideal approaches to improve the quality of the emotional eating. Researchers contend this is one motivation behind why yoga is so amazing—due to the accentuation on the breath. It encourages us to unwind by initiating the emotional eating and supporting our sensory system. Slow stomach breathing can improve vagal tone. Likewise, Ocean-Sounding Breath (Ujjayi pranayama), in which you make a delicate narrowing in the back of your throat, can additionally upgrade the advantages. The emotional eating contacts the throat, so making a tad of rubbing in the throat as you inhale can help invigorate the vagus and improve vagal tone. Have a go at delaying during work to inhale profoundly for a couple of seconds, and notice how you feel.

❖   **EXERCISE**

Moderate to concentrated exercise has been appeared to improve pulse inconstancy, the marker of vagal tone. Studies show that normal exercise in sound grown-ups, just as grown-ups with cardiovascular illness, improved vagal tone. The exercise doesn't need to be long-only 20 minutes can have an effect. While look into this has not yet been done, it would appear to pursue that consolidating yogic breathing with moderate exercise would additionally upgrade the impacts of pressure versatility and vagal tone.

❖   **METTA MEDITATION**

Metta reflection, otherwise called cherishing thoughtfulness contemplation, is simply the act of sending kind considerations to yourself as well as other people. Scientist Barbara Fredrickson found that Metta's contemplation improved vagal tone for some who rehearsed it. She contrasted a control bunch with those rehearsing Metta and found that when individuals revealed increments in warm and cherishing sentiments, their vagal tone improved. Have a go at rehearsing Metta contemplation as you nod off; not exclusively will you improve your vagal tone, you may likewise be emphatically affecting your fantasy life, as per the Buddhist writings.

❖   **BRIEF RECITATION**

An examination demonstrated that reciting on can improve vagal tone by invigorating the nerves around the throat. On the off chance that isn't your thing, you can likewise have a go at singing noisily— what the hell, nobody's tuning in the vehicle. Feel the reverberation in your throat and all through your body.

Plainly yoga offers an assortment of apparatuses to increment vagal tone and along these lines bolster pressure flexibility. The key is to rehearse at least one of these instruments every day, regardless of whether it's only for five minutes. Also, recall, it sets aside an effort to fortify the sensory system, yet persistence and practice can carry us to a progressively adjusted condition of being.

The emotional eating is really a basket case driving from the gut through the heart and to the cerebrum. It's the longest cranial nerve and has correspondence with each organ.

Its fundamental capacity is to control the parasympathetic sensory system. The parasympathetic sensory system is a piece of the autonomic help framework known as the "rest and overview" framework. It assumes a job in pulse, sexual excitement, absorption, pee, and gastrointestinal action.

The emotional eating works enthusiastically to control irritation. It alarms the cerebrum to discharge synapses when provocative proteins called cytokines are available. These synapses help the body fix at that point decrease aggravation.

Another capacity of the emotional eating is to trigger the arrival of acetylcholine which controls muscles, enlarges veins, and eases back pulse. It's sheltered to state the emotional eating might be the most significant nerve that most of the individuals are as yet ignorant of.

Researchers have connected emotional eating brokenness to heftiness, constant aggravation, wretchedness, uneasiness, seizures, unusually low pulse, blacking out, and GI issues.

Actually, the examination on this nerve has been promising to the point that emotional eating triggers have been embedded in patients and discovered achievement even with untreatable sadness and epilepsy. The gadget is carefully embedded under the skin and sends an electrical sign to the emotional eating. When invigorated, the emotional eating begins speaking with the remainder of the body.

Fortunate for us, there's no requirement for a medical procedures. Vagal tone can be improved normally through incitement with systems that should be possible at home. Attempting to reinforce your vagal tone will help with state of mind, processing, and general prosperity.

Nineteen Efficient Ways To Improve Emotional Eating

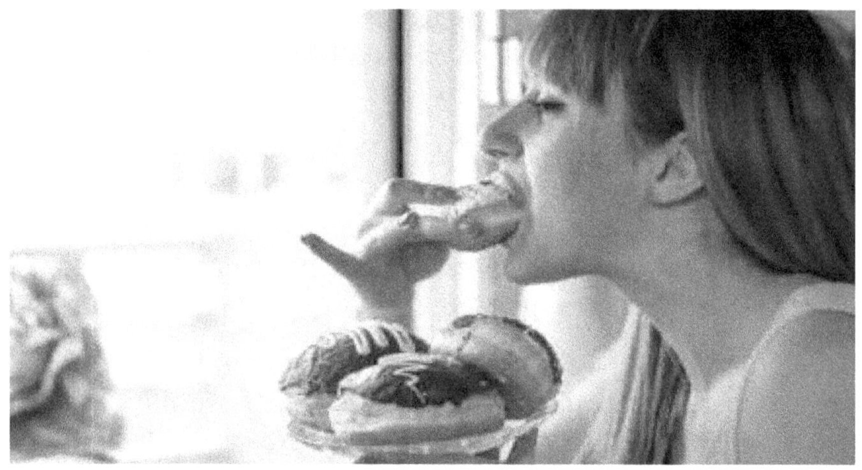

1. SWISHING. This is presumably the least complex and most open route for an individual to chip away at their vagal tone. In the first part of the day wash some water as hard as possible. You'll realize you've invigorated the emotional eating when you start to get a tear reaction in your eyes.

2. BREATHWORK. Profoun d moderate breaths from the tummy will animate the emotional eating. Sit or set down and take in as much as you can. Hold it for a second or two and afterward discharge. Rehash this 5-10 times. You'll feel euphoric and lose a while later.

3. GIGGLING. Giggling discharges a huge amount of synapse which improves vagal tone. Giggle hard and regularly.

4. FISH OILS. EPA and EHA lower pulse which reinforces vagal tone.

5. FASTING. The emotional eating is the chief of the parasympathetic sensory system known as the rest and condensation framework. Offering the assimilation procedure a reprieve through discontinuous fasting or fewer snacks for the duration of the day will likewise improve vagal tone.

6. YOGA. The breathing and development of yoga assist with absorption and has been appeared to build GABA levels. Improving GABA levels will animate the vagal tone.

7. SINGING. Singing works the muscles in the back of the throat which invigorates the emotional eating. Simply make certain to sing as loud as possible for this impact to occur. An extraordinary spot to do this is in the vehicle.

8. COLD SHOWERS. Cold showers are extreme from the start, yet they can enormously improve vagal tone. As you change in accordance with the cool, the thoughtful sensory system brings down and the parasympathetic framework gets more grounded legitimately influencing the emotional eating.

9. BACKRUB. A back rub invigorates the lymphatics and improves the vagal tone.

10. FRAGRANCE BASED TREATMENT. Fundamental oils, for example, lavender and bergamot have appeared to expand pulse inconstancy which improves vagal tone.

11. DEVELOPING POSITIVE RELATIONSHIPS. Research shows that just by thinking about our friends and family we can tone and reinforce the emotional eating, consequently receiving the numerous rewards that the nerve gives.

12. PRESENTATION TO THE COLD. By drinking cold water or washing up, we reinforce our body's quieting framework (the parasympathetic framework) which occurs through the emotional eating.

13. SINGING AND CHANTING. Singing as loud as possible expands pulse inconstancy and works the muscles in the back of your throat that associate with the emotional eating.

14. BACK RUBS. Apart from feeling astounding, a great back rub of the feet and neck actives the emotional eating and can diminish seizures.

15. SATISFACTION AND LAUGHTER. Having a decent snicker lifts your mind-set, supports the insusceptible framework and animates the emotional eating.

16. YOGA AND TAI CHI. Both Yoga and Tai Chi give a large group of medical advantages and are especially useful for those battling with wretchedness and nervousness.

17. PROFOUND BREATHING. Profound breathing animates the emotional eating to bring down circulatory strain and pulse.

18. EXERCISE. Physical exercise is ground-breaking both for gut stream and psychological well-being benefits, which both happen by means of the emotional eating.

19. UNWINDING. Practically any loosening up action reinforces the vegas nerve's capacity to give recuperating to the body.

Therefore, These Are Ways That Can Help Strengthen The Vagal Tone For You.

You may need to quit taking certain drugs early, and your PCP may ask you not to eat the night prior to the system.

❖   **WHAT YOU CAN ANTICIPATE**

Prior to a medical procedure, your PCP will do a physical assessment. You may require blood tests or different tests to ensure you don't have any wellbeing worries that may be an issue. Your primary care physician may have you start taking anti-microbial before medical procedures to avoid disease.

❖   **DURING THE TECHNIQUE**

Medical procedure to embed the emotional eating incitement gadget should be possible on an outpatient premise; however, a few specialists suggest remaining medium-term.

The medical procedure, for the most part, takes an hour to 90 minutes. You may stay conscious yet have drugs to numb the medical procedure territory (nearby anesthesia), or you might be oblivious during the medical procedure (general anesthesia).

The medical procedure itself doesn't include your mind. Two cuts are made, one on your chest or in the armpit (auxiliary) district, and the other on the left half of the neck.

The beat generator is embedded in the upper left half of your chest. The gadget is intended to be a perpetual embed, however, it tends to be expelled if important.

The beat generator is about the size of a stopwatch and runs on battery control. A lead wire is associated with the heartbeat generator. The lead wire is guided under your skin from your chest up to your neck, where it's appended to one side emotional eating during that time entry point.

❖   **AFTER THE METHODOLOGY**

The beat generator is turned on during a visit to your primary care physician's office half a month after a medical procedure. At that point it very well may be customized to convey electrical motivations to the emotional eating at different terms, frequencies, and flows. Emotional eating incitement, for the most part, begins at a low level and is slowly expanded, contingent upon your indications and reactions.

Incitement is customized to turn on and off in explicit cycles —, for example, 30 seconds on, five minutes off. You may make them shiver sensations or slight genuine annoyance and transitory dryness when the nerve incitement is on.

The trigger doesn't recognize seizure action or melancholy side effects. At the point when it's turned on, the trigger turns on and off at the interims chose by your PCP. You can utilize a hand-held magnet to start incitement at an alternate time, for instance, in the event that you sense a looming seizure.

The magnet can likewise be utilized to incidentally kill the emotional eating incitement, which might be essential when you do certain exercises, for example, open talking, singing or working out, or when you're eating in the event that you have gulping issues.

You'll have to visit your primary care physician occasionally to ensure that the beat generator is working accurately and that it hasn't moved out of position. Check with your primary care physician before having any restorative tests, for example, attractive reverberation imaging (MRI), which may meddle with your gadget.

❖　　**RESULTS**

Embedded emotional eating incitement isn't a solution for epilepsy. A great many people with epilepsy won't quit having seizures or taking epilepsy medicine inside and out after the methodology. However, many will have fewer seizures, up to 20 to 50 percent less. Seizure force may diminish too.

It can take months or even a year or longer of incitement before you see any critical decrease in seizures. Emotional eating incitement may likewise abbreviate the recuperation time after a seizure. Individuals who've had emotional eating incitement to treat epilepsy may likewise encounter upgrades in disposition and personal satisfaction.

Sooner or later, we have all experienced obstruction. It's awkward, irritating, and can frequently demonstrate agonizing. In addition, if not took care of, it can prompt an affected colon, which might be deadly.

In instances of obstruction, it's enticing to just reach for a jug of purgatives to explain the issue. However this solitary treats the side effect not the reason.

Frequently, blockage is an aftereffect of not being adequately hydrated. On the off chance that you haven't been expending enough water, the body accepts each accessible open door to build its very own stores—including taking it from nourishment.

In a condition of parchedness, the colon will endeavor to separate water from anything you have devoured, abandoning a hard remainder—what will in the long run become your stool. With little water content, it's currently dry and unallowable, making it hard to go through the colon as well as the inside. The outcome: obstruction.

Moreover, salivation (which we will take a gander at in more detail presently) is the principal phase of assimilation. It starts by separating the nourishment to make a structure which would then be able to be effectively prepared by the colon. Inadequate hydration implies less salivation and along these lines an expanded remaining burden for the remainder of your body.

So to stay customary, drink water. It's without a doubt desirable over taking medicine to calm the issue.

Only a snappy expression of counsel. Clogging can likewise be a side effect of a progressively genuine fundamental issue. In case you're experiencing this infirmity regularly, counsel with a medicinal expert.

Medical advantages of water

❖   **HELPS YOU LOSE WEIGHT**

I know numerous individuals who effectively decrease their water admission when attempting to get thinner—this can be a serious mix-up.

Their hypothesis is that any overabundance water devoured will be held and along these lines lead to weight gain. However by and large, that is an error.

The facts confirm that feminine cycle or certain illnesses, for example, kidney infection and heart issues, can prompt inordinate water maintenance. Be that as it may, these are the consequences of different issues—not drinking a lot of water.

The truth of the matter is water can really advance weight reduction. **Here's the ticket.**

Giving a Feeling of Fullness

Research has shown that expending water alongside your suppers expands the sentiment of satiety. This implies you're more averse to eat an enormous part, return for quite a long time, or have a treat.

This can decrease the admission of pointless calories that lead to weight gain.

- **Raising The Metabolic Rate**

Drinking water has appeared to increment thermo genesis—the raising of inside internal heat level.

As the body heats up, the metabolic rate is raised, pushing all its compound responses and procedures into overdrive. This state requires vitality (calories) to fuel the expansion in digestion, which can be found in your fat stores.

- **Can Reduce Caloric Intake**

One of the principle explanations for weight gain, or the powerlessness to get in shape, is the utilization of calories. In the event that admission surpasses consumption, you put on the pounds.

While numerous individuals effectively screen their nourishment admission, what's frequently disregarded is the quantity of calories that beverages give. For instance, a standard jar of pop contains around 140 calories, while an enormous mocha espresso from an outstanding chain indicates 420 calories for every cup.

Drinking water as a substitution to soft drinks and sweet smooth espressos expel a surprisingly high number of calories from the eating routine (water is without calorie). Be that as it may, on the off chance that regardless you need that caffeine hit, settle on a dark

Americano—made for the most part from water with no milk and, in this manner, zero calories.

❖   **PREVENTS THE ONSET OF HANGOVERS**

The terrible sentiments related with an aftereffect—cerebral pain, annoyed stomach, and exhaustion—are normally the side effects of a certain something: lack of hydration.

Liquor causes you to lose water—it's a diuretic. It might create the impression that you are taking in fluids, however you're really losing them. Normally, the most ideal approach to stay away from aftereffects isn't to drink liquor, yet in certain conditions, it's neither alluring nor commonsense.

The way to balance the opportunity of an aftereffect is to expend a lot of water. There are differing suppositions on the ideal method for accomplishing this.

One of the most mainstream is to drink a sizeable measure of water—around 16 to 18 ounces—before rest, which ought to supplant any liquor actuated water misfortune.

In any case, my undisputed top choice is to switch among liquor and water during drinking periods. That is, after each mixed drink, expend a glass of water. This has two constructive outcomes.

To begin with, it replaces liquids lost because of the diuretic impact of liquor. Second, it can really make you drink less, as water makes you feel full.

❖   **PROMOTES HEALTHY KIDNEYS**

Kidneys are astounding at detoxifying the body. They gather together all the destructive components you've expended and remove them before they arrive at hazardous levels.

The issue is the point at which you don't expend enough water—

you're putting extreme weight on this fundamental pair of organs.

One of the most significant issues that can happen is kidney stones. These are developments of mineral gems which cluster together, hindering the kidney's capacity or inciting torment as they go down and become stopped in the ureter or urethra.

Expending adequate water can forestall kidney stone arrangement. The more water that goes through the kidneys, the simpler the removed minerals are to flush out—before they can shape into stones.

❖   **ENHANCES BRAIN POWER**

The cerebrum is around 75 percent water. So any kind of lack of hydration quickly influences its constitution and capacity.

The positive advantages of expending water for the mind are various, including:

- Improved state of mind

- Improved transient memory

- Raised readiness

- Supported intellectual capacity

A decent method to kick-start the mind each day is to begin your morning schedule with a glass of water. During rest, we lose a ton of this component through sweat, inward compound procedures, and relaxing.

Recharging these stores following waking will give the mind the underlying lift it needs to control you as the day progressed.

❖   **INCREASES PHYSICAL PERFORMANCE**

In the case of practicing at home or partaking in aggressive games, staying hydrated is basic to keep execution at ideal levels.

It's nothing unexpected that being physically dynamic uses our water stores, particularly when pushing hard and along these lines losing extreme water through sweat.

Be that as it may, it's not only enough to renew these stores once the activity has wrapped up. To remain continually in top structure, hydration is required during the physical effort itself. Indeed, even little misfortunes of water (under two percent of volume) can weaken execution. The purpose behind this is water is an indispensable piece of numerous procedures associated with physical effort.

One of the primary regions is that of muscle compression, the demonstration required in each physical exercise (and in every day schedules). Water upgrades the intensity of the muscle-building proteins, gives versatility and quality, transports minerals, gives vitality, and supplies the muscle-controlling adenosine triphosphate (ATP).

So guaranteeing that we are adequately hydrated implies that muscles are attempting to most extreme limit.

Being dried out, in any case, can genuinely diminish our presentation yield:

Decreasing blood stream fundamental for shipping oxygen and supplements

Debilitating heart capacity and bringing down circulatory strain, diminishing vitality yield and productivity

Bringing down the viability of glycogen put away in the muscles with water

Expanding the development of lactic corrosive, which brings down both stamina and continuance

Advancing muscle breakdown rather than development by

decreasing testosterone and raising cortisol levels

❖   **KEEPS HEADACHES AT BAY**

We frequently credit our cerebral pains to pressure, noisy commotion, or only a part of human life that must be acknowledged. Ordinarily, it brings about us gulping several painkillers and afterward attempting to continue ahead with our day.

The issue is once in a while, particularly on account of headaches, they can be crippling and in excess of a unimportant irritation. However as a rule, this could basically be brought about by not devouring enough water.

Evidence shows cerebral pains and headaches can be initiated by lack of hydration. What's considerably all the more intriguing is a similar writing states that expending water once the agony has begun reduces the side effects—without the utilization of medicine.

Why We Get Food Cravings

There is some contention about precisely why we get desires. A few specialists propose that the pestering aches are physiological. Our bodies long for specific supplements when we need the outcome that the nourishment may bring. For instance, a treat gives a sugar surge. Or then again we may desire comfort nourishments as an approach to expand sentiments of solace.

There are additionally hormones associated with appetite and desires. Researchers realize that lepton, ghrelin and different hormones in your body can change the manner in which we experience hunger. Analysts are attempting to see how and in the event that they can change hormones to assist calorie counters with managing desires and yearning.

In any case, different specialists state desires are essentially a component of propensity. For instance, we may nibble on nourishment when we are exhausted or when we are searching for an approach to maintain a strategic distance from work that we need to do.

Furthermore, wellness and wellbeing specialists frequently disclose to us that nourishment yearnings can happen when our bodies are got dried out.

So which clarification is the genuine answer? It's conceivable that nourishment desires are brought about by a mix of both physiological and situational factors. It is additionally conceivable that various health food nuts are influenced by various causes.

5 Ways To Bust Food Cravings

Knowing the reason for your yearnings may assist you with quieting the inclination to eat when you're on an eating routine. Be that as it may, there are different approaches to oversee nourishment desires to get thinner.

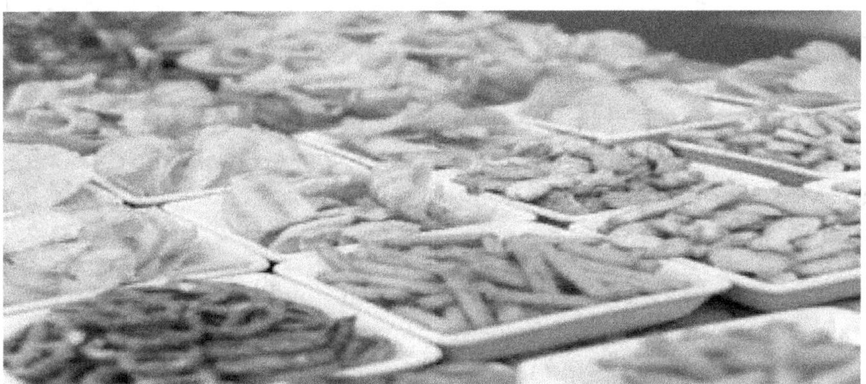

❖   **TRY NOT TO GO ON A VERY LOW-CALORIE DIET**

In the event that you're eating routine is excessively low in calories, you're probably going to have nourishment yearnings that are too difficult to even consider managing. At the point when you following a severe arrangement, it feels like you are being denied. In certain individuals, this prompts gorging or surrendering their program totally.

Rather, pursue a solid low-calorie feast plan that takes into consideration some incidental treats. By settling on better decisions and having periodic treats, your longings are probably going to diminish.

Basic Printable Meal Plans to Help You Lose Weight.

❖　　**CHEAT (HOWEVER ONLY A BIT)**

You can't eat carrots to fulfill a hankering for carrot cake. Now and then, when you're truly longing for something, you simply need to eat it. Be that as it may, you can do as such that keeps your eating routine on track. Set aside a few calories in your week by week calorie spending plan and have a little treat as a reward. By eating only a tad of the nourishment you're truly pining for, you'll manage the nourishment longing for head-on and possibly avoid indulging.

❖　　**OCCUPY YOURSELF**

There are a few days when it appears as though the nourishment you desire is all over the place. Maybe a collaborator carries doughnuts to the workplace or perhaps you pass your preferred drive-through eatery while in transit to the red center. It very well may be difficult to oversee nourishment fixation when you're looked with your preferred food sources each day.

You can't keep away from the nourishment totally; however you can make a redirection so you don't see it to such an extent. On the off chance that doughnuts are in the workplace lunchroom, at that point have a solid lunch in a close by café and maintain a strategic distance from the lounge inside and out. In the event that you pass your preferred low quality nourishment joint while in transit to the rec center, discover another course that causes less pressure.

❖　　**FIGURE OUT HOW TO IDENTIFY AND MANAGE EMOTIONS**

Desires aren't generally the aftereffect of feelings, however for a few of us, there's no denying the association. We eat when we are focused or dismal or encountering tension.

On the off chance that you eat in light of your emotions, you have to deal with your sentiments first and afterward handle the nourishment yearnings. Why? Since nibbling on your preferred treat won't recuperate passionate agony. Try not to be hesitant to request help in the event that you experience these issues. Weight reduction can pause, however your passionate prosperity must be a need.

❖   **ENDURE IT**

In all honesty, now and then the most ideal approach to manage nourishment yearnings is to coarseness your teeth and endures it. On the off chance that you essentially overlook it and proceed onward, it might vanish. In the event that you can persuade yourself it's brain over issue, you may discover desires aren't such a considerable rival after all!

Desires for things like cabbage or child carrots are uncommon (and in the event that you have them, I salute you). Rather, desires are for the most part for nourishments high in fat, sugar, or carbs (hi, chocolate secured pretzels!) which, when ingested, trigger the arrival of characteristic narcotics and give us a feeling of delight—a sort of scaled down high. In reality, zones of the mind related with sedate longing for light up when individuals ache for particular nourishment. Moreover, blocking sedative receptors in the cerebrum cuts yearnings for fat and sugar.

Hormones assume a job in yearnings, as well. Ghrelin, the craving hormone, normally goes here and there when a feast. In any case, developmentally, ghrelin is as yet living on the fields from our chasing and assembling days—it assumes a job in our common inclination for sugar, just as our probability of surrendering to desires for comfort nourishments.

Ghrelin may likewise shield us from halting at only one serving of Chubby Hubby: A recent report found that ghrelin levels pursued a run of the mill rise-and-fall design in the wake of eating a moderately exhausting feast, yet soared off the diagrams subsequent to eating yummy heavenliness (explicitly, cake with rum syrup, custard, and Nutella) much after the investigation members were full.

This recommends ghrelin drives what analysts call "epicurean nourishment utilization," which is what's going on when your chocolate croissant feels suspiciously like baked good wrapped break. In a hormonal one-two punch, eating for delight additionally obliged diminished degrees of the hormone that impacts satiety. This may have been useful in past centuries, however isn't useful when you work over the road from Krispy Kreme.

Eating to fulfill a hankering is not the same as a gorge. Yearnings can set off a gorge, yet they don't need to. A gorge feels wild and is regularly determined by pressure, stress, disgrace, or fatigue. It is regularly, yet not generally, related with utilizing nourishment to fill an enthusiastic void or overseeing apparently unmanageable feelings.

Longings, on the other hand, aren't really determined by feeling; however they can get stirred up with them. Desiring for particular nourishment frequently goes connected at the hip with different sentiments, and comprehending what you're managing is the initial step to avoidance. With that in mind, here are

4 Scoundrels Garments Of Desires:

❖   EMOTIONAL EATING

Enthusiastic eating is additionally called pressure eating. The two longings and passionate eating mirror a powerful urge, yet with a hankering, the object of want is the particular nourishment—you need something exceptionally specific and alternate nourishment won't work. On the other hand, the purpose of enthusiastic eating is just the demonstration of eating, regardless of whether to consume apprehensive vitality, relieve yourself, or stuff a sentiment of vacancy. Particular nourishment may be liked, yet any nourishment will do, as Oprah's celebrated occurrence with solidified frank buns and syrup bears witness to.

❖   **BOREDOM**

In case you're an animal of propensity, eating similar nourishments throughout each and every day may be a solace. In any case, for the individuals who improve assortment, limiting yourself to nourishments that are natural or advantageous lights a fire under yearnings. An investigation in the diary Physiology and Behavior found that "dietary dullness," in any event, when it meets every single healthful need, triggers yearnings. This regularly happens to calorie counters; people on an eating routine frequently eat a similar hardly any things in light of the fact that the nourishments are "allowable" or they definitely know the caloric substance. This can prompt weariness, which can trigger a hankering.

❖   **DEPRIVATION**

By a similar token, weight watchers frequently deny "awful" nourishments. Be that as it may, refusing certain nourishments works like idea concealment, or, in other words it doesn't. For instance, make an effort not to consider a pink elephant coasting over your head. Try not to stress—I can't do it, either. Presently, do whatever it takes not to consider steak frites. Since you need to recollect what shouldn't think about—or what shouldn't eat—it's consistently at the forefront of your thoughts.

On the off chance that you feel denied when you attempt to aggregate nourishments as "solid" versus "unfortunate" or "great" versus "awful," you might be setting yourself up for yearnings. Eat what you like in reasonable sums, before the feeling of hardship develops.

The enormous bullet to this announcement is that for a few, the forbearance model truly works best. In the event that you can't eat only one Oreo without setting off a Cookie Monster free-for-all, and you're OK with never having them in the house, essentially don't get them. Your life will be simpler for it.

❖ PLAIN OLD HUNGER

On the off chance that it's been in excess of a couple of hours since you've eaten, it probably won't be a hankering, as such, yet straightforward yearning. The distinction: hunger is fulfilled by numerous nourishments, while a hankering is squelched by one specific nourishment. So if everything in the shop case looks great, you're most likely simply eager. Additionally, a hankering in the end passes, however hunger just deteriorates. So feed yourself. What's more, in case you're eager for something explicit, appreciate.

❖ REMEMBER A HANKERING ISN'T A CRISIS

As opposed to getting cleared up in the criticalness of "I need it presently!" let the hankering roost on your shoulder and bear it for some time. Like a tempest, longings fail and pass. Welcome it as a transitory guest instead of battling it like an adversary.

❖ LEAN IN

To oppose the hankering, utilize an outlandish apparatus and incline toward the hankering. Your body may require affirmation and consideration, not Fritos. Relax. Tranquilly see and depict the hankering in unromantic terms. You may reveal some other need under the hankering, or you may not; it's the tuning in that will let you know.

❖ DELAY

A few yearnings resemble a sparkler—a fast pop and they break up. Be that as it may, others are a moderate consume—they seethe on for quite a long time and days if not satisfied. To manage the sparkler assortment, reveal to yourself you can have that salt and vinegar potato contributes thirty minutes. Quick forward to your objective time and you may have disregarded them. In the event that despite everything you need them, possibly you have the moderate consume.

Into the shopping basket they go, however do the accompanying:

Ladies, work it out; respectable men, hush up about it. A recent report found that when ladies attempted to stifle their considerations about chocolate, they really wound up eating half more than the individuals who were urged to ponder it. For men, in any case, the reaction was unique—the individuals who contemplated the chocolate wound up eating more than the individuals who smothered.

❖ **DON'T ATTEMPT TO SUBSTITUTE OR THEN AGAIN FOUR**

I'm willing to wager you're comparative. In case you need something, don't attempt to trick yourself. Your body and taste buds are savvy, and they will get distraught on the off chance that you attempt to deceive them.

❖ **CREATE A SMALL SCALE CUSTOM FOR YOUR PREFERRED NOURISHMENTS**

Taking part in custom around nourishment makes it increasingly agreeable. Lighting candles, singing "Upbeat Birthday," and making a desire truly improves. Be that as it may, it chips away at a littler scale, as well. In a recent report from the University of Minnesota, something as little as opening a chocolate bar with a particular goal in mind made the members appreciate the chocolate longer, rate it all the more profoundly, and pay more for it. Do likewise and make a custom around nourishments you hunger for to augment your happiness. You don't need to do a detailed doughnut move; it could be as straightforward as continually breaking the doughnut down the middle before you eat it.

❖ **SAVOR IT**

At the point when you at last get your hands on that pot corn, truly taste it. Eat it gradually. Sit at a table, yet not before a screen. Bite, don't breathe in. Taste every fixing. This is called careful eating and it very well may be both liberating and disappointing. The propensity to drive through a feast without tasting it is regular to such an extent that it feels odd to back off, yet eating carefully can diminish your longings, your waistline, and your danger of Type 2 Diabetes. However, not to stress—your nourishment doesn't need to be extravagant, vegetarian, or natural—you can eat anything carefully, even your children's pizza hulls (not so I know anything about that...)

CHAPTER 13

LEARN WHAT IS THE NEGATIVE SELF-TALK

❖ **SELF-SABOTAGE**

Apart from people who suffer from food-related body conditions, many people indulge is self-negative talk. It is a form of self-sabotage as it prevents you from seeing the best out of yourself or from making decisions that will make your life and health better.

Negative self-talk is looking down upon or undermining yourself and losing belief in your ability to wholeness. It is all about hating oneself.

People who engage in negative self-talk make a big deal out of small situations that could either be overlooked or solved in a short period. For example, after overeating in a party, a self-sabotaging person will dwell on it and feel bad enough to cause the rise of stress hormones which may lead to further overeating.

A self-sabotaging person also tends to make everything they hear personal. They are paranoid about everything. They could be at a conference that addresses issues related to obesity and they will feel like the speaker was addressing them personally or speaking about their weaknesses. They always feel attacked. This may lead to people isolating themselves, which is a symptom that may lead to depression.

People who engage in negative self-talk possess the 'I can't' mentality. They do not believe they can make a change in their habits or weaknesses even if they need to. They cannot influence people, they look down on themselves.

These people also feel helpless. They feel like they cannot be anything other than what they believe they already are. These people could be at the best of their health and still belittle themselves and feel unhealthy. They might not be conscious of their being.

People who engage in negative self-talk suffer from stress, depression and low self-esteem.

❖ TO OVERCOME SELF-SABOTAGE

People who engage in negative self-talk must surround themselves with positive people. This will allow them to see wellness in themselves and appreciate themselves.

It is also good that they realize their selves, their potential and be positive about it, lower their expectations on how people treat them or on what to expect from people. This will give them a higher chance to work on their inner selves, not to feel disappointed or feeling unworthy before others.

Self-sabotages must also learn to deal with their attitude. They must be self-conscious and intentional about their attitude so that they can control how they feel about themselves.

They must believe in themselves. For anyone else to value who you are, they must first believe that you value yourself. It is only a person who can determine how others look at him or her.

Smiling and saying thank you take one a long way. It causes the mind to feel positive and creates a positive attitude that is important to boost the confidence of people who engage in negative self-talk.

Exercising the body also rejuvenates the mind and causes good feelings that are important for people who look down on themselves. Engaging in family activities also helps!

CHAPTER 14

I'M NOT ON A DIET

I Recollect The First Run Through The Idea Flew Into My Brain:

"I am fat! "

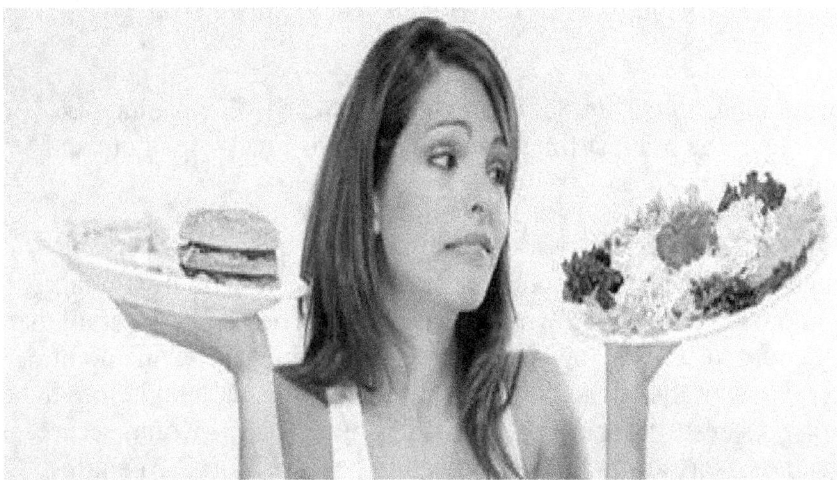

I was 12 years of age. There were such a large number of things I didn't think about my body. However, I made certain in a certain something, I have to get thinner. It was summer and I was wearing dark shorts and a white T-shirt. I glanced myself in the mirror and felt something that would later turn out to be so well-known — being awkward in my own skin.

I was 12 and reluctant.

Rather than not having a consideration on the planet, I began turning out to be increasingly more fixated on my body. As years passed, my self-perception turned out to be much increasingly contorted. I was 14 when I finished up my best alternative is to quit eating. I would eat as much as I have to endure the day. On better days it was a banana.

After some time, I understood it is difficult to work this way. It was critical to me to be acceptable at school. At the point when I understood I didn't have the vitality to learn or to think, I chose I expected to change something. "I must eat to have vitality, yet I likewise frantically need to lose weight." so I concluded I would gobble and afterward make myself hurl.

Around then, I knew nothing about anorexia or bulimia nervosa or that such a large number of individuals feel the manner in which I do.

I began rehashing a similar example consistently. Eat as much as Possible in the briefest time conceivable until I feel wiped out and afterward hurl.

Before long my folks saw I was acting abnormally. They separated from a couple of years sooner and we were living with my mother. My mom acknowledged what was going on. They had a go at all that they could to support me. We went to see a clinician. At the point when I was in the latrine, my poor mother was remaining before the entryways ensuring that I don't hurl. From the start, I would secure myself in the restroom and attempted to be as peaceful as could reasonably be expected. She took the key out. I began to stand by longer after I wrapped gobbling and afterward hurl in my room. She was keeping an eye on me constant when she wasn't grinding away.

I was fortunate that my folks saw what was going on.

I was additionally fortunate to acknowledge on time that I would make myself wiped out, perhaps irreversibly, on the off chance that I precede down that street.

So I quit doing it consistently. I did it now and again. After some time I was doing it less and less. There were times when I wouldn't do it for a considerable length of time. At that point some way or another, I quit doing it totally.

At the point when I put it that way, it sounds so natural. It was difficult. I was battling each day. On one side there was that sensible piece of me that was revealing to me I have to stop or I would genuinely hurt my wellbeing. On the opposite side, there was the nauseate I felt for the manner in which I looked, for the manner in which I felt and the sentiment of absolute vulnerability.

Despite the fact that I didn't starve myself any longer and I quit hurling after my dinners, thinking designs that drove me to it remained with me for a long, long time.

Now and again I sensed that I was in a war with myself.

I needed to spare myself, and yet, I was unable to quit being the cause all my own problems.

I was battling with myself, crying and asking whatever it is, to disregard me so I could carry on with my life. I needed to feel free. Appreciate life.

Nourishment was the focal point of my musings. My days spun around what I should eat, when should I eat, what is and isn't permitted and battling against the desire to voraciously consume food and hurl.

I was in an endless loop and I was unable to get out. Needing to eat something yet not permitting myself — eating a little piece trusting that I won't feel regretful — feeling blame and nauseate — rebuffing myself.

My method for discipline? Eating all that I considered unfortunate that I could discover/have at that point. Sentiments of disgrace, misery and blame that followed that scene were my greatest discipline.

This proceeded for quite a long time. During that time, I was continually attempting to calculate my purposes for it. I was attempting to support myself. At this time, I feel good saying that I succeeded.

What's Stowing Away Underneath The Surface?

At the point when you're 12, you aren't totally ready to comprehend for what reason are a few things occurring. For what reason do I have the considerations I have?

For what reason wouldn't i be able to eat nourishment like every other person, appreciate it without feeling regretful about it?

For what reason is it unimaginable for me to take a bit of sweets, eat a frozen yogurt or a cake and proceed with my day?

Rather, on the off chance that I ate a bit of treats, I would be so frustrated and feel such significant sicken for myself that I would rebuff myself by pigging out until I felt disgrace, blame and self-detest. "You are so frail. Presently eat until you feel sick."

It was the most noticeably awful discipline for me, not just on account of my dread of gaining weight yet in addition as a result of the emotions and considerations that followed.

I was wrecking myself, harming myself such that I knew would be intellectually generally excruciating to me. What's more, I accepted that I merit it.

As I was getting more seasoned, particularly when I entered school, I began chipping away at myself. I needed to become acquainted with myself, comprehend my contemplations and activities and above all, comprehend what is activating them.

I began watching my contemplations.

I gradually understood that I don't have issues with nourishment, I have issues with myself.

Nourishment was just the instrument I utilized for my wound prize and discipline framework.

There are a wide range of elements that may add to building up a dietary problem. One such mental factor is an inclination of deficiency or absence of control throughout everyday life.

At the point when I was 12 years of age, my folks separated. Indeed, even before their separation, I knew there was unfaithfulness on the two sides (I felt something was wrong, been nosey and discovered things). Both of my folks had new accomplices not long after the separation. Despite the fact that around then I didn't feel that I was very disturbed and harmed, I presently accept these occasions assumed a significant job in my conduct. All that I knew and adored was changing and will never be the equivalent. Sentiment of losing control, joined with my hairsplitting, affectability, compassion and the need to shield my more youthful sibling from being harmed and simultaneously realizing that I was unable to support him, was simply a lot for me.

Outwardly, I was an upbeat little youngster, extraordinary at school, incredible at sport, having a ton of companions, ready to do anything. Within, I was self-destructing. I felt frail, deficient and powerless. I would not like to feel like that, I was embarrassed about it. So I went to self-discipline. I expected to recover the control. What's more, I felt in charge when I controlled my eating. At the point when I had the option to avoid nourishment and get thinner I felt solid and pleased. At the point when I was unable to oppose some nourishment, I was powerless and defenseless once more, and I would rebuff myself with all the more eating and additionally languishing.

That dread of insufficiency, not being sufficient and negative self-discernment is something I have conveyed with me into adulthood. Be that as it may, when I had the option to comprehend myself I realized I was on a way to recuperation.

I had terrible days, when I would slip into pointless conduct once more. I had not really awful days when I just had negative considerations, however not followed by voraciously consuming food, hurling or limiting myself nourishment.

Be that as it may, I additionally had incredible days, when I delighted in nourishment without blame.

Program Your Mind To Slim Body

On the off chance that you have ever attempted to get fit, you realize that eating well nourishment and moving your body are significant parts of any weight reduction plan. Be that as it may, did you realize that coming to or keeping up a solid body creation occurs in both your body and your psyche? Truth be told, in the event that you have attempted over and over to get thinner yet have never been effective or you get thinner yet then restore it (to say the very least!), almost certainly, your contemplations and convictions—not your eating regimen—are keeping you down.

That is on the grounds that overabundance weight is an impression of your psychological or enthusiastic state. What's more, the main explanation individuals neglect to get in shape is that they disregard to make changes in their subliminal psyche to help their cognizant objectives.

I've gone through over 45 years contemplating nourishment and its consequences for ladies' bodies, psyches, and spirits—both by and by and expertly. Being brought into the world with a body that my folks named "strong," I've needed to work deliberately on tolerating my size and weight for the greater part of my life. Also, having worked with a large number of ladies with a similar issue, I can guarantee you that I realize what works and what doesn't.

❖   **HOW YOUR BELIEFS CAN THWART YOUR WEIGHT-LOSS EFFORTS**

Ladies get negative messages about their bodies for their entire lives. It's no big surprise that the eating regimen business is blasting. With an ever increasing number of individuals going to diets, exercise, and contrivances to control their weight, it's an easy decision that eats less carbs simply don't work. However numerous ladies attempt to get in shape quickly, frequently before going to an exceptional occasion, for example, a wedding, school gathering, or get-away. Be that as it may, right around 90 percent of the time, they recapture the weight in light of the fact that the arrangement was not practical. In this way, these ladies build up the constraining conviction that they will always be unable to get thinner or keep up their ideal weight.

Other basic constraining convictions that can shield you from accomplishing your weight and body size objectives frequently originate from dread. For instance, on the off chance that you were explicitly manhandled when you were more youthful, you may expect that, in the event that you get more fit, others will discover you alluring and hurt you explicitly. Or then again maybe you are anxious about the possibility that that in the event that you get more fit at the same time, at that point don't discover an accomplice, you will be viewed as a disappointment. A few people clutch weight out of the dread that more will be normal from them once they are slender. Others may expect that in the event that they get fit, they will be dismissed by their family or companions. There is additionally the regular dread that on the off chance that you aren't "the hefty individual," you won't know what your identity is.

The explanation these convictions are constraining is on the grounds that, so as to discharge undesirable weight, your cognizant and subliminal personalities must concur. On the off chance that your brain says, "I need to get more fit, and I trust I can do so effectively," and your subliminal psyche concurs, you will get fit. In any case, if your subliminal brain believes that you will always be unable to accomplish your ideal weight, you will no doubt battle to shed pounds regardless of your cognizant want.

❖　　　**THE MOST EFFECTIVE METHOD TO RESHAPE YOUR BODY WITH YOUR THOUGHTS**

Accepting you don't have a metabolic issue or clinical issue keeping you from arriving at your weight reduction objectives, the initial step to shedding pounds is to turn out to be intensely mindful of your story. This might be the account of your past, for example, a relative continually squeezing your midriff and calling you "chubs." Or it might be a later story that you started letting yourself know. For instance, you may over and again disclose to yourself that weight reduction is hard a result of your powerlessness to eat right and exercise because of the extended periods you spend grinding away.

Keep in mind, your considerations and convictions make your existence. Thus, before endeavoring to change your eating routine and exercise schedule, it's a smart thought to chip away at changing your considerations and convictions.

Here Are 12 Practices For Reconstructing Your Intuitive To Accomplish Lasting Weight Reduction:

Tune in to your self-talk. Sense of pride and self-acknowledgment are the foundations to accomplishing ideal weight. Be that as it may, a great many people can't shed pounds since they participate in body-disgracing talk and conduct. It's critical to realize how you've been conversing with yourself before you attempt to get more fit. On the off chance that you have been telling your body that you loathe what it looks like for an amazing majority or squeezing your skin in the mirror in appall on the grounds that somebody used to do this to you, your subliminal brain will accept the negative programming. By conversing with your body in a positive, adoring way—the manner in which you would address a **blameless kid**—you can overhaul your intuitive cerebrum. Glance in the mirror and distinguish what you love about your body. Contact the parts that you need to change and state, "Thank you for guarding me." Assure your body that it is protected to shed pounds. Do this consistently. After some time, your intuitive will line up with your cognizant want to shed pounds.

Compose another story. Rather than trying to say you need to get more fit, record precisely what you need to accomplish and why. Possibly you need to shed 5 pounds (or 50 pounds) so you can stay aware of your grandkids. Or on the other hand possibly you need to settle on better nourishment decisions with the goal that you have more vitality. Make certain to record how you feel now and how you will feel when you accomplish your objectives.

For instance, if being overweight shields you from getting a charge out of bicycle rides with your companions and this cause you to feel forgot about, record this particular circumstance and feeling. At that point record how you will feel when you lose the additional pounds and can participate in the good times. As you begin to reveal your feelings around arriving at your weight objectives, keep on thinking of them down. Make certain to recount to your new story to yourself consistently. Let it saturate your subliminal and each cell in your body.

Take a stab at Tapping. Tapping, or the Emotional Freedom Technique (EFT), assists with adjusting your intuitive psyche to your objectives on a vivacious level by tending to the hidden feelings, designs, convictions, injuries, and more that can prompt weight gain. You start by expressing your present restricting conviction followed by expressing how you cherish and acknowledge yourself while tapping on explicit pressure point massage focuses.

For instance, you can say, "Despite the fact that I make some hard memories shedding pounds, I cherish and acknowledge myself totally." This decreases pressure hormones in your body and assists with discharging the passionate recollections and convictions related with the undesirable pounds so you can get out from under old propensities and mend. (Figure out how to play out a tapping arrangement here.)

Contemplate. Reflection is another instrument that can assist you with getting progressively mindful of your contemplations and convictions so you can cut a way to fruitful weight reduction. You can utilize your reflection practice to reveal your inspirations for needing to get in shape, see any passionate or intuitive squares, and even use symbolism of how shedding pounds may look and feel to decidedly overhaul your cerebrum and grow more sympathy for yourself. On the off chance that sitting in contemplation isn't your thing, take a stab at moving reflection, for example, yoga or Qigong. You may likewise like tuning in to sound reflections, for example, the free contemplations from the Center for Mindful Eating.

Set supportable objectives. Your definitive objective might be to shed 80 pounds, however in case you're set on accomplishing that immediately, you might be setting yourself up for disappointment.

Rather, set littler, practical objectives. For instance, start with objectives you have command over, for example, eating 5 servings of foods grown from the ground every day or remaining hydrated by drinking (and eating) more water. You can likewise set an objective to get 8 hours of rest for each night.

You may find that these supportable objectives alone assist you with getting thinner. On the off chance that you need to set a real weight reduction objective, ensure it's close to 2 pounds for each month. I realize this sounds low, however 2 pounds for every month is reasonable, and in 1 year that adds up to 24 pounds!

Eat carefully. Studies show that care—concentrated consciousness of your considerations, activities, and inspirations—assumes a fundamental job in long haul weight reduction when utilized with other weight reduction systems. Practice care as you approach setting up your dinners and eating. Attempt to be aware of sentiments of appetite and totality. Focus on tastes, surfaces, and the demonstrations of biting and gulping your nourishment. Likewise, be aware of how your body feels after you eat certain nourishments.

This training can help lessen gorging and make you increasingly mindful of propensities that don't bolster your weight reduction objectives. At the point when you begin interfacing what you eat with how you believe, you won't have to eat less carbs to get in shape. It will happen easily. At the point when you change your disposition about nourishment as self-sustenance, your body sythesis, and self-perception will likewise be changed. At the point when you interface with your body and support it from a position of sympathy and sense of pride, the sentiments related with that dignity make a metabolic milieu in your body that is helpful for ideal fat consuming.

State assertions. Certifications help to strengthen the new story you are customizing your intuitive to accept. They function admirably when they are authentic. Be that as it may, on the off chance that you state, "I will be 80 pounds lighter in one month," your subliminal will have a hard time believing it. Rather, take a stab at saying, "I'm turning into the normally thin individual who lives within me!" Or state, "I presently settle on solid choices that help my ideal weight."

You can even make a custom of saying your certifications. For instance, you can smear your room or home of dormant vitality, light a flame, sit with your eyes shut, and state your assertions multiple times in succession.

Do this 2 or 3 times each day. You might need to state some variant of your certifications not long before you nod off when your subliminal psyche is generally open to recommendation. Keep in mind, assertions should be in the current state as if they have just showed. In the expressions of Michael Beckwith of the Agape Church, "Assertions don't get something going. They make something welcome."

Diet Is Not Obligation, It's A Choice For My Health

The dangers of poor nourishment

Great nourishment, in view of good dieting is one basic factor that encourages us to remain sound and be dynamic.

❖ **WHAT CAUSES POOR NOURISHMENT**

Poor dietary patterns incorporate under-or over-eating, not having enough of the sound nourishments we need every day, or devouring an excessive number of sorts of nourishment and drink, which are low in fiber or high in fat, salt or potentially sugar.

These undesirable dietary patterns can influence our supplement consumption, including vitality (or kilojoules) protein, starches, basic unsaturated fats, nutrients and minerals just as fiber and liquid.

❖ **HOW DOES POOR SUSTENANCE INFLUENCE US**

Poor sustenance can disable our every day wellbeing and prosperity and decrease our capacity to lead an agreeable and dynamic life.

For the time being, poor nourishment can add to pressure, tiredness and our ability to work, and after some time, it can add to the danger of building up certain diseases and other medical issues, for example.

- Being overweight or hefty
- Tooth rot
- Hypertension
- Elevated cholesterol
- Coronary illness and stroke

Type-2 Diabetes

- Osteoporosis
- A few malignant growths
- Wretchedness
- Dietary problems.

Steps to great sustenance - it's simpler than you might suspect

A decent spot to begin is to:

Have a decent assortment of solid nourishments from the five nutrition classes every day. For more data see the Healthy eating for various ages and organizes and Healthy Eating tips areas

- Focus on two serves of leafy foods serves of vegetables every day
- Just sometimes eat sugary, greasy or salty nourishment, and afterward just in modest quantities
- Drink new, clean faucet water rather than sugary beverages
- switch over to sound plans that look and taste great
- Prepare and look for sound fixings
- Appreciate preparing and eating well nourishment with family or companions and without interruptions, for example, the TV.

CONCLUSION

Passionate eating. The name practically summarizes it: eating in light of negative feelings like pressure, uneasiness, pity, and so on. Narrative, it's a quite regular event. In the event that you remained on a city intersection reviewing passersby, all things considered, most would underwrite every so often striking the pantry for something sweet or salty (or both) following an exhausting day at the workplace.

Be that as it may, in the exploration world, there are two camps rising with regards to passionate eating. More or less, a few people believe it's a thing, and others believe it's definitely not.

Having done a reasonable piece of research on the subject (see my 2017 article for a full survey of the connection between passionate eating and weight results), I've seen a strong group of proof to help the legitimacy of enthusiastic eating. At the point when individuals take a gander at the connection between passionate eating and weight after some time, as anyone might expect, they will in general locate that enthusiastic eaters put on more weight than non-passionate eaters. Passionate eaters don't simply tend to gain weight; they likewise experience more prominent challenges taking it off.

With regards to conduct weight reduction mediations (frequently alluded to as RCTs or randomized controlled preliminaries in look into), enthusiastic eaters additionally lose less weight than the individuals who don't take part in passionate eating. What's more, it is anything but a unimportant sum either. When seeing all out weight reduction as far as the level of starting body weight lost, enthusiastic eaters lose around 4 percent not exactly non-passionate eaters.

Given that 5 percent weight reduction is sufficient to esteem it clinically noteworthy; implying that it assists with diminishing the hazard for other wellbeing concerns like diabetes, coronary illness, and other interminable intricacies, 4 percent is an entirely huge number. In light of the entirety of this current, it's anything but difficult to make the determination that passionate eating isn't only a "thing" that individuals do every now and then, but instead a conduct that has genuine ramifications for long haul wellbeing and prosperity.

So regardless of these discoveries, for what reason do others contend against passionate eating? Furthermore, what elective clarification do they give? Given that the assortment of writing on enthusiastic eating is huge, the examination done on overweight and corpulent people depicted above is just a subset of the entirety of the investigations done right now. There is additionally a genuinely exhaustive measure of research on ordinary weight people also.

In these examinations, ordinary weight individuals (which from an institutionalized perspective normally alludes to those inside a to some degree self-assertive BMI scope of 18.5-24.9, in spite of the fact that the benefits of BMI for portraying weight warrant their own article for one more day), as a rule undergrad college understudies, participate in lab contemplates taking a gander at passionate eating.

Normally, they experience a state of mind enlistment, which includes viewing a tragic video, or tuning in to dismal music, to set them feeling negative, and afterward they are offered an assortment of nourishments to look over and their utilization is estimated. Taking a gander at these sorts of studies, the discoveries are blended with regards to whether negative feelings really lead to expanded nourishment consumption.

It's hard to make any strong determinations since specialists in each camp have their contentions against the contrary side. One of the confinements to the ordinary weight considers is that they are for the most part genuinely imagined. Placing somebody in a research center investigation and watching their conduct isn't really demonstrative of what you would find in their everyday life. That being stated, the inquiry despite everything stays with regards to why some ordinary weight people evidently participate in enthusiastic eating yet figure out how to keep up their weight. There are several distinct hypotheses on this.

One is that typical weight people basically misattribute their gorging to their feelings. Since passionate eating is such a well known social build, it's anything but difficult to eat a lot of something and afterward state, "Goodness, I did that since I was very worried." There is some proof to show that when individuals gorge, they tend to accuse negative feelings sometime later as a simple out to represent why they ate more than they believed they ought to have.

Another hypothesis is that typical passionate eaters are simply greater at automatic than overweight and fat enthusiastic eaters. They may take part in precisely the same conduct, however do it to a lesser degree and utilize different instruments to adapt. For instance, they may eat in light of negative feelings, yet at the same time stop when they are full, and furthermore do customary exercise to keep up their way of life.